Cornea

ESASO Course Series

Vol. 6

Series Editors

F. Bandello Milan
B. Corcóstegui Barcelona

Cornea

Volume Editor

José L. Güell Barcelona

85 figures, 81 in color, and 9 tables, 2015

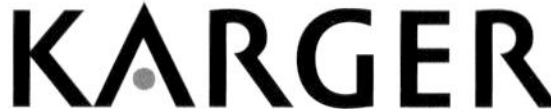

Basel · Freiburg · Paris · London · New York · Chennai · New Delhi ·
Bangkok · Beijing · Shanghai · Tokyo · Kuala Lumpur · Singapore · Sydney

José L. Güell
IMO. Instituto Microcirugia Ocular of Barcelona
Autonoma University of Barcelona
C/ Josep Mª Lladó, 3
ES–08035 Barcelona (Spain)

Library of Congress Cataloging-in-Publication Data

Cornea (Güell)
Cornea / volume editor, José L. Güell.
     p. ; cm. -- (ESASO course series, ISSN 1664-882X ; vol. 6)
  Includes bibliographical references and index.
  ISBN 978-3-318-05452-1 (hard cover : alk. paper) -- ISBN 978-3-318-05453-8
(e-ISBN)
  I. Güell, José L., 1960- , editor. II. European School for Advanced
Studies in Ophthalmology, issuing body. III. Title. IV. Series: ESASO course
series ; v. 6. 1664-882X
  [DNLM: 1. Cornea--surgery. 2. Refractive Surgical Procedures. WW 220]
  RE336
  617.7'19059--dc23
                                          2015018826

Bibliographic Indices. This publication is listed in bibliographic services, including Current Contents®.

© Copyright 2015 by S. Karger AG, P.O. Box, CH-4009 Basel (Switzerland)
www.karger.com
Printed in Germany on acid-free and non-aging paper (ISO 9706) by Kraft Druck, Ettlingen
ISSN 1664–882X
e-ISSN 1664–8838
ISBN 978–3–318–05452–1
e-ISBN 978–3–318–05453–8

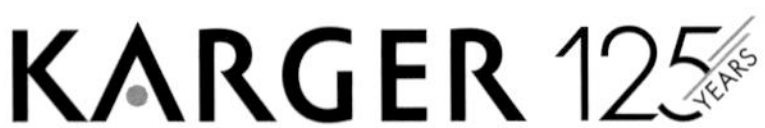

Contents

List of Contributors

Myriam Cassagne
Department of Ophthalmology, Purpan Hospital
1 place du Dr Baylac
FR–31059 Toulouse (France)
E-Mail cassagne.m@chu-toulouse.fr

Harminder S. Dua
Academic Ophthalmology Section, Division of
Clinical Neuroscience
University of Nottingham
Nottingham BG7 2UH (UK)
E-Mail profdua@gmail.com

Safa El Hout
Department of Ophthalmology, Purpan Hospital
1 place du Dr Baylac
FR–31059 Toulouse (France)
E-Mail nadinehout@hotmail.com

Mostafa El Husseiny
Research Institute of Ophthalmology
2 Al Ahram
Giza (Egypt)
E-Mail mostafahus@hotmail.com

Thomas A. Fuchsluger
Department of Ophthalmology
University of Erlangen-Nürnberg
Schwabachanlage 6
DE–91054 Erlangen (Germany)
E-Mail thomas.fuchsluger@uk-erlangen.de

Oscar Gris
Instituto Microcirugia Ocular of Barcelona
c/ Josep Mª Lladi 3
ES–08035 Barcelona (Spain)
E-Mail gris@imo.es

José L. Güell
IMO. Instituto Microcirugia Ocular of Barcelona
Autonoma University of Barcelona
C/ Josep Mª Lladó, 3
ES–08035 Barcelona (Spain)
E-Mail guell@imo.es

Soraya M.R. Jonker
University Eye Clinic Maastricht, Maastricht University
Medical Center
P. Debyelaan 25
NL–6202 AZ, Maastricht (The Netherlands)
E-Mail soraya.jonker@mumc.nl

Friedrich E. Kruse
Department of Ophthalmology
University of Erlangen-Nürnberg
Schwabachanlage 6
DE–91054 Erlangen (Germany)
E-Mail friedrich.kruse@uk-erlangen.de

George D. Kymionis
Vardinoyiannion Eye Institute of Crete (VEIC)
University of Crete, Faculty of Medicine
GR–71003 Heraklion, Crete (Greece)
E-Mail kymionis@med.uoc.gr

François Malecaze
Department of Ophthalmology, Purpan Hospital
1 place du Dr Baylac
FR–31059 Toulouse (France)
E-Mail malecaze.fr@chu-toulouse.fr

Felicidad Manero
IMO. Instituto Microcirugia Ocular of Barcelona
C/ Josep Mª Lladó, 3
ES–08035 Barcelona (Spain)
E-Mail manero@imo.es

Leonardo Mastropasqua
Ophthalmology Clinic, Centre of Excellence in
Ophthalmology, National High-Tech Eye Center (CNAT)
University 'G. d'Annunzio' of Chieti-Pescara
Via dei Vestini
IT–66100 Chieti (Italy)
E-Mail mastropa@unich.it

Morral Merce
Hospital Clínic i Provincial de Barcelona
ES–08036 Barcelona (Spain)
E-Mail merce.morral@gmail.com

Mario Nubile
Ophthalmology Clinic, Centre of Excellence in
Ophthalmology, National High-Tech Eye Center (CNAT)
University 'G. d'Annunzio' of Chieti-Pescara
Via dei Vestini
IT–66100 Chieti (Italy)
E-Mail m.nubile@unich.it

Rudy M.M.A. Nuijts
University Eye Clinic Maastricht, Maastricht University
Medical Center
P. Debyelaan 25
NL–6202 AZ, Maastricht (The Netherlands)
E-Mail rudy.nuijts@mumc.nl

Isabelle E.Y. Saelens
University Eye Clinic Maastricht, Maastricht University
Medical Center
P. Debyelaan 25
NL–6202 AZ, Maastricht (The Netherlands)
E-Mail isabelle.saelens@mumc.nl

Dalia G. Said
Department of Ophthalmology, Queens Medical
Centre, University Hospital
Nottingham NG7 2UH (UK)
E-Mail daliagsaid@yahoo.com

Caterina Sarnicola
University of Ferrara
Via Savonarola, 9
IT–44121 Ferrara (Italy)
E-Mail c.sarnicola@hotmail.it

Enrica Sarnicola
University of Siena
Via Mazzini n°62
IT–58100 Grosseto (Italy)
E-Mail e.sarnicola@hotmail.it

Vincenzo Sarnicola
Ambulatorio di Chirurgia Oculare Santa Lucia
Via Mazzini n°62
IT–58100 Grosseto (Italy)
E-Mail v.sarnicola@hotmail.it

Preface

Today, there are multiple attractive options for postgraduate training in ophthalmology, but at the same time, these are frequently confusing for the surgeon: which is the best option to select, taking into account the time and space limitations that we all need to deal with? We can focus on peer-reviewed journals and papers, specialized books, national and international meetings and courses, multiple specialized as well as more general websites, etc., all of them useful but with their own particular limitations: sometimes these are already a little bit 'outdated' or disorganized when they reach our desk; sometimes we have some inconvenience to attend the proper meetings; and, on other occasions, we have low scientific and academic support. This is why some European societies are strongly focusing on investing time and resources on education as their main goal, as is the case for the European Society of Cataract and Refractive Surgeons (ESCRS) and the European Society of Cornea and Ocular Surface Disease Specialist (EuCornea).

Based on our experience and an excellent response from the participants in teaching modules in Lugano, the main goal of the ESASO Book Series has been to offer the ophthalmology trainee an up-to-date review of a selection of important topics, mixing basic information with the most advanced techniques. In this book, the individuals responsible for each lesson are corneal and ocular surface surgeons as well as refractive surgery specialists who are well known worldwide and who have invested a significant amount of their time in generously teaching and sharing their own experience with academics. We hope that you will enjoy this first volume on a selection of topics on corneal surgery and corneal refractive procedures.

Jose L. Güell, MD, Barcelona

Güell JL (ed): Cornea. ESASO Course Series. Basel, Karger, 2015, vol 6, pp 1–25
DOI: 10.1159/000381489

The Ocular Surface: Functional Anatomy, Medical and Surgical Management

Harminder S. Dua[a, b] · Dalia G. Said[b]

[a] Academic Ophthalmology Section, Division of Clinical Neuroscience, University of Nottingham and [b] Queens Medical Centre, University Hospital, Nottingham, UK

Abstract

The ocular surface (OS) is a functional unit comprising the eyelids and blink reflexes, tear film and tear glands, the conjunctival mucus membrane and substantia propria, and the corneal epithelium and Bowman's zone. Its health is crucial for vision. The OS can be affected by a variety of degenerative, inflammatory and neoplastic diseases, as well as by trauma. Significant amongst these are dry eye disease, microbial infections and immune-mediated inflammatory disorders ranging from allergic conjunctivitis to destructive conditions such as ocular cicatricial pemphigoid and chemical burns. Several of these can lead to persistent epithelial defects with risk of perforation. Management principles include a thorough history and clinical evaluation of signs and symptoms to establish the diagnosis and determine the extent of disease. Treatment is tailored to the specific condition and ranges from lubricant drops to antimicrobial agents and anti-inflammatory drugs such as steroids and steroid-sparing agents. A variety of surgical procedures are often required both as adjunctive or primary interventions. These can be simple outpatient procedures such as punctal plugs and tarsorrhaphy or complex procedures such as amniotic membrane grafts, keratoplasty and limbal stem cell transplantation. In end-stage diseases where the OS is severely compromised and dry, keratoprosthesis remains the only hope to restore some sight.

The Ocular Surface

The term 'ocular surface' (OS) was coined by Richard Thoft [1] to include the entire mucus membrane lining from the lid margins across the posterior surfaces of the eyelids, the superior, inferior, medial and lateral fornices, the eye ball, the limbus and the corneal surface together with the tear film. As an anatomical unit, the OS includes the entire conjunctival, the limbal and corneal epithelium. However, as a functional unit, the OS includes the eyelids and their movements together with the glands that secrete the various components of the tear film. As far as the depth of the OS is concerned, different authors have been fairly liberal in limiting it to the epithelium or extending it to the entire thickness of the conjunctiva and all layers of the cornea.

Functional Anatomy

The key player at the OS is the transparent cornea, which interfaces with light rays as they traverse to the retina. The other elements of the OS serve to maintain a healthy environment in which the cornea can retain its transparency and facilitate vision. Despite its very organized structure, the epithelium of the cornea is a poor optical surface without the 'polish' provided by the tear film.

Tear Film and Conjunctiva
This is a dynamic complex structure that is served by numerous cells and glands and that is continuously replenished and evenly distributed across the OS by the blinking action of the eyelids. The tears are primarily made of mucin derived from the epithelial cells and goblet cells of the conjunctiva, an aqueous component derived from the lacrimal and accessory lacrimal glands and an oil component derived from the meibomian glands of the eyelids. The hydrophobic surface of the corneal epithelium is rendered hydrophilic by the binding of mucin to the epithelial cells. This allows the aqueous component to form a relatively thick layer on the mucin bed, upon which the meibomian oil (meibum) spreads as a thin layer, delaying both evaporation and the breakup of the tear film. Though the tear film is described as a trilaminar structure, it is now known that the three laminae are not distinct and defined; instead, a gradient of mucin admixes with the aqueous component from the epithelium to the oil layer. In addition, the tears contain a myriad of proteins, growth factors, vitamins, electrolytes and a few cells that collectively contribute to the nourishment, defence and health of the OS [2].

In the interest of transparency, the cornea has to forsake an established blood supply, which is restricted to the limbal arcades. The cornea therefore relies on nutrients provided via the aqueous humour, the tear film and the limbal vessels. Oxygen from the atmosphere dissolved in the tear film reaches the cornea; hence, contact lenses can potentially interfere with this process and cause adverse consequences. Equally noxious agents such as carbon monoxide from smoke can also dissolve in tears and reach the cornea. The exposed position of the eyes renders the cornea especially vulnerable to injury and to microbial invasion from the environment [3]. Immunoglobulins, lysozyme, lactoferrin and a number of antimicrobial peptides provide innate defence, which is backed up by cell-mediated and humoral responses by the resident and circulating lymphocytes of the conjunctival mucosal immune system. The conjunctival substantia propria is known to express many high endothelial venules during inflammation to facilitate exit of mononuclear cells, and even to demonstrate follicular aggregations with germinal centres. This enables the conjunctiva to respond to a number of different insults, which in turn, can compromise its health. Conjunctival health determines corneal health [4].

The importance of the tears cannot be overestimated. Dry eyes cause troublesome symptoms and blurring of vision and considerably affect the quality of life of the patient. Many interventions to restore sight involve the transplantation of tissues such as corneal, limbal and amniotic membrane (AM) tissue. No living tissue transplant can survive for long in a dry environment.

The Limbus
The microanatomy of the limbus reveals a defined stromal architecture with a unique blood supply, the palisades of Vogt, the interpalisade rete ridges, and the limbal epithelial crypts. Collectively, they provide the anatomical basis and the physiological microenvironment for the maintenance of corneal epithelial stem cells (SCs). The physiological turnover of the corneal epithelium throughout life requires new cells to take the place of those that are lost. This is facilitated by the limbus, which acts as a repository of SCs [5]. Though there is some evidence that the basal epithelium of the cornea (transient amplifying cells) can sustain the physiological demand, there is no doubt that in response to injury or insult, limbal SCs play an important role in regenerating the corneal surface [6]. Features of the normal and deficient/abnormal limbus have been defined clinically and by in vivo confocal microscopy. The palisade architecture is maintained in the

Fig. 1. Diffuse slit lamp image of limbal palisades of Vogt. Pigmented palisades are easy to visualise. The linear palisades (**a** and **b**) and the rounded accessory palisades seen at the conjunctival (**a**) and corneal (**b**) aspects of the linear palisades are clearly visible. The palisades and interpalisade rete ridges are repositories of stem cells.

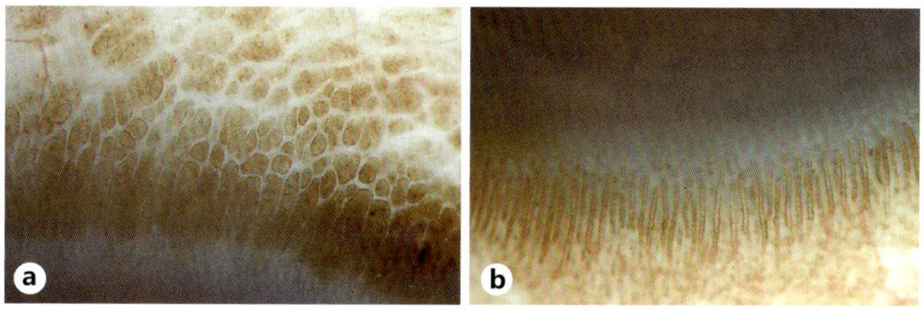

stroma underlying the basal cells, and limbal epithelial crypts are often particularly detectable in pigmented palisades, where confocal visibility is better [7–10] (fig. 1a, b).

Often, a large part of the central corneal epithelium can be lost whilst a rim of peripheral and limbal epithelium survives. This is due to the enhanced adhesion of peripheral/limbal basal cells to the underlying basement membrane, which allows these cells to survive and function to resurface the cornea. Such injuries to the corneal epithelium that retain an intact limbus heal via the formation of 2–6 centripetally migrating convex-fronted epithelial sheets that meet each other along adjacent surfaces, giving the defect a geometric shape (triangular, quadrilateral, pentagonal, or hexagonal), which eventually closes via the formation of Y-shaped contact lines that are visualized by fluorescein stain and represent the pseudodendrites associated with the healing of corneal abrasions (fig. 2a). In injuries in which the limbus is affected, healing occurs via the circumferential migration of tongue-shaped epithelial sheets that arise from each end of the surviving epithelium (usually in the upper half). These migrate along the denuded limbus until they meet. Thereafter, the defect behaves like one with an intact limbus following the same sequence as described above (fig. 2b). In some instances, the centripetally migrating conjunctival epithelium of the adjacent conjunctival defect can encroach on the denuded limbus and cornea, resulting in conjunctivalization of the

cornea. This is considered as a hallmark of limbal SC deficiency (LSCD) [11–13] (fig. 2c).

Established concepts related to SC are now challenged by emerging clinical situations such as surviving central islands of epithelial cells in the presence of total LSCD [6] and by the transdifferentiation of the conjunctival epithelium into a corneal phenotype on the corneal surface. Mesenchymal SCs that have been shown in specific sites such as foetal liver, bone marrow and dental pulp have also been demonstrated in the corneal stroma. These cells have immense potential for clinical use for tissue regeneration.

Corneal Innervation

The principal nerve supply comes from the ophthalmic division of the trigeminal nerve via the long posterior ciliary nerves. These nerves arborize posterior to the limbus and form a perilimbal plexus from which nerves enter the cornea radially in equal numbers all around (approximately 11 per quadrant). These divide and subdivide as stromal nerves, predominantly in the anterior two thirds of the cornea, and move anteriorly to a sub-Bowman's plexus, from which smaller branches penetrate Bowman's membrane and end in two to six small bulbs per nerve. The majority of nerves penetrate Bowman's membrane outside the central 5 mm zone of the cornea. From the bulb-like structures finer, neurites emerge to form the sub-basal plexus (fig. 3), from which terminal nerve endings enter the epithelium and demonstrate both inter- and

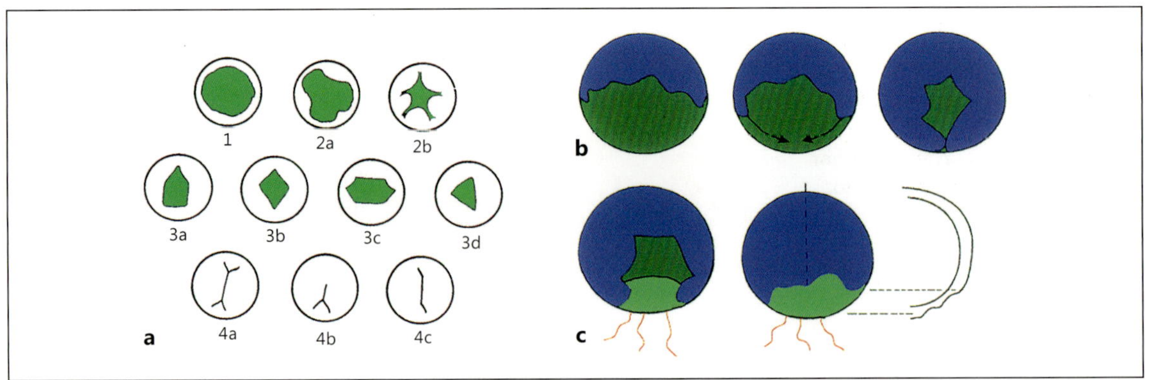

Fig. 2. a Diagrammatic representation of a healing corneal epithelial wound with an intact limbus. A circular defect (1) heals by the formation of up to 6 convex-fronted sheets of epithelium from the limbus (2a, 2b). Adjacent sheets meet and undergo contact inhibition to form geometric shapes (triangular, quadrilateral, pentagonal, or hexagonal (3a–3d)). These eventually close with the formation of Y-shaped contact lines that can be incomplete and can appear as 'pseudodendrites' (4a–4c). (Reproduced from author's publication [12].) **b** Diagrammatic representation of a healing corneal epithelial wound with involvement of the limbus. Two tongue-shaped sheets of epithelium arise from each end of the remaining intact limbal epithelium (left) and migrate circumferentially (middle) until they meet each other, affording complete cover to the limbus (right). After limbal healing is complete, the central defect follows the pattern as described in **a** above. (Reproduced from author's publication [55].) **c** Diagrammatic representation of the migration of the conjunctival epithelium onto the cornea when the limbus is involved. The conjunctival epithelium crosses the limbus (left) to cover a variable area of the cornea (middle). This results in limbal stem cell deficiency, and the area attracts blood vessels, has an irregular surface (right) and shows delayed fluorescein staining. (Reproduced from the author's publication [13].)

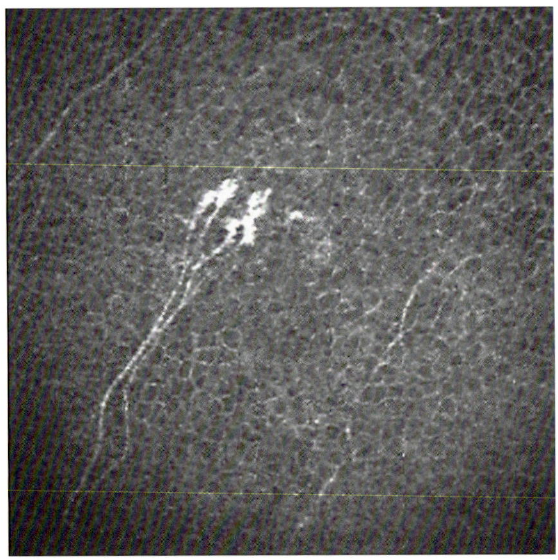

Fig. 3. In vivo confocal image of two subepithelial terminal bulbs from which neurites are seen to arise. These contribute to the corneal sub-basal nerve plexus.

intracellular terminations. The nerves serve sensory, trophic and vasomotor functions. The limbal vascular arcade responds to corneal nerve stimuli via vasodilation (circumcorneal congestion) and diapedesis of white blood cells (triple response), which invade the cornea to combat noxious and infective agents. In situations in which innervation is compromised, infective organisms can flourish in the absence of the host response in a unique pattern of infection called infectious crystalline keratopathy [14, 15].

A large number of diseases affect the function and or structure of the OS. Diseases can be inflammatory – infective (virus, bacteria, fungi, protozoa, or parasites) or non-infective – chronic, subacute, acute, immune-mediated – hypersensitivity (allergic) cell-mediated – degenerative, neoplastic, traumatic (surgical) or congenital (aniridia and dystrophies).

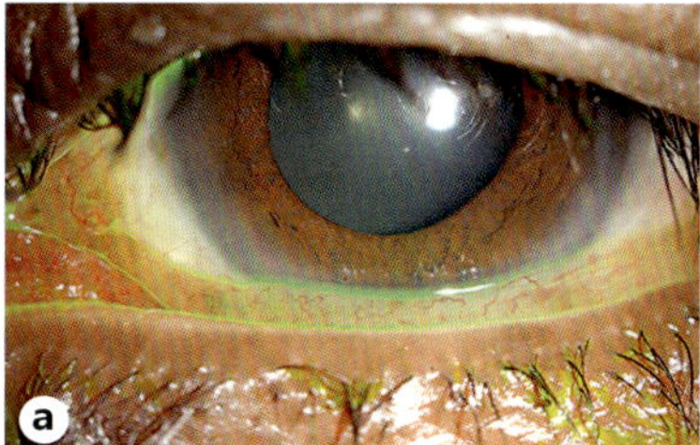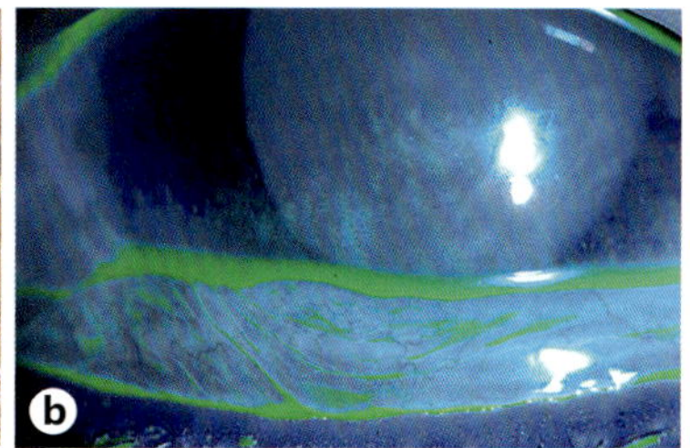

Fig. 4. a Inferior conjunctival chalasis. **b** Note the tear distribution on the surface and at the superior edge of the chalasis. The inferior cornea shows punctate erosions due to tear distribution problems.

Principles of Management

Dry Eye

Definitions

An international panel met in Baltimore in 2004 and, by adopting the Delphi approach, introduced the term dysfunctional tear syndrome (DTS) to describe dry eyes. They concluded that DTS can be present with or without clinically evident inflammation and with or without reduced tear volume with an associated alteration in tear composition [16]. This definition incorporates the suggestion that dry eye symptoms can occur when tear volume is normal but when tear distribution is altered, as is the case for conjunctival chalasis or surface lesions (fig. 4a, b).

The following year, the Dry Eye Workshop produced a comprehensive definition of dry eye: a multifactorial disease of the tears and the OS that results in symptoms of discomfort, visual disturbance, and tear film instability, potentially resulting in damage to the OS. Dry eye is accompanied by increased osmolarity of the tear film and inflammation of the OS [17]. Importantly, both definitions incorporate the term 'inflammation' into the pathogenesis of dry eye.

Patients with dry eye disease or DTS often present with complaints of sore or gritty eyes, which can be worse upon waking. Women are almost twice as likely to suffer as men, and the severity is exacerbated after menopause. The approach to management is determined by the symptoms, signs and underlying pathology. Ag-

gravating factors such as car heating, air travel, computer use, and excessive use of hair dryers can be addressed. Computers have become an integral part of modern day life style. Hot air that emanates from computers and accessory devices such as printers can create an envelope of warm air in the immediate environment of the user (personal observation). This environment, coupled with the reduced blinking associated with near work can trigger or worsen symptoms. The use of alternative medication or the cessation of medication for patients on drugs that cause dry eye, such as antihistamines, tricyclic antidepressants, and selective serotonin reuptake inhibitors, should be considered [18].

Other measures include limiting or discontinuing the use of contact lenses, stopping smoking, avoiding smoky atmospheres, and using humidifiers. Special measures are needed for treating blepharitis associated with dry eye. These include lid hygiene with lid-cleansing wipes, heat treatment, which can be dry (e.g. Eyebag) or moist (e.g. Blephasteam goggles) (fig. 5), lid massage with a warm wet hand towel or sophisticated devices (e.g. Lipiflow) and the use of oral tetracycline or topical azithromycin [19, 20]; these two antibiotics help to contain commensal flora that might flourish in dry eye states and decrease the production of bacterial lipase, thus reducing the amount of free fatty acids that can affect the lipid composition of the tear film. They also have anti-collagenase activity and an anti-chemotactic effect on neutrophils.

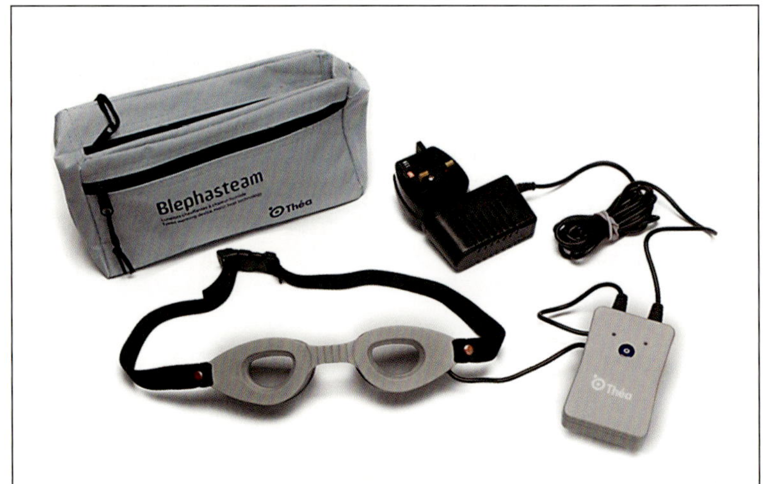

Fig. 5. Blephasteam (Thea®). This spectacle-type device provides moist heat to the eyes and eyelids and helps in the management of meibomitis. (The authors have no financial interest to declare with regard to this device.)

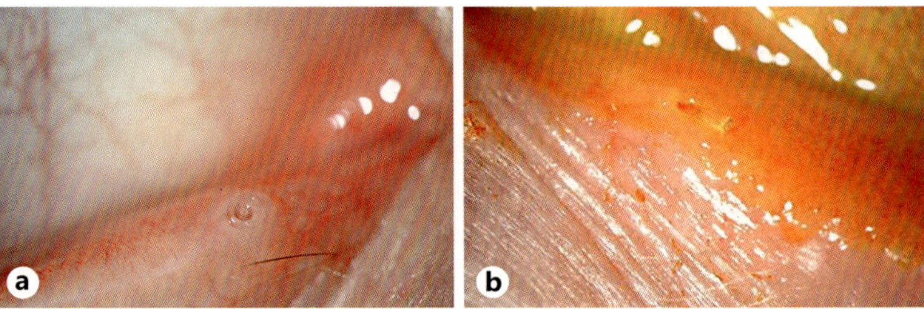

Fig. 6. a Punctal plug in situ in the lower punctum. **b** A canalicular plug (Smart plug) is inserted into the canaliculus. It slowly disappears into the canaliculus as the long slender rod shrinks at body temperature into a short and thickened plug.

Clinical assessment of dry eye includes, besides a thorough history and eye examination, specific tests for tear function, namely Schirmer's test, tear film break-up time, tear meniscus height, fluorescein dye clearance and tear osmolarity. For most tests, there is considerable overlap between the normal and abnormal ranges (symptomatic patients may have normal values, and asymptomatic patients may have abnormal values), but increased tear osmolarity is considered a fairly specific indicator of dry eye.

These patients should be made to understand that the condition may not be cured but that symptoms can be relieved or alleviated and that there are likely to be good days and bad days. Artificial tear drops are the mainstay in the management of dry eye symptoms. A wide range of artificial tears is available, and the list is ever growing. One approach is to start with the simplest (cheapest) and work one's way through the list until the patient finds one that suits him/her the best. Tear substitutes are used for symptomatic relief of dry eyes. They are hypotonic or isotonic buffered solutions, and they differ in their osmolarity, viscosity, electrolyte composition and preservatives. Most artificial tear drops contain preservatives such as benzylkonium. This compound is fairly toxic to the OS and can aggravate the dry eye condition. Preservative-free drops are of benefit in patients who have to use eye drops very frequently or for a long period of time [21]. Newer tear substitutes are designed to reduce osmolarity and either avoid the use of preservatives or contain preservatives that disintegrate on contact with the eye. In some patients, the use of punctal (fig. 6a) or canalicular plugs (fig. 6b) can reduce the need or frequency of instillation of tear drops [22].

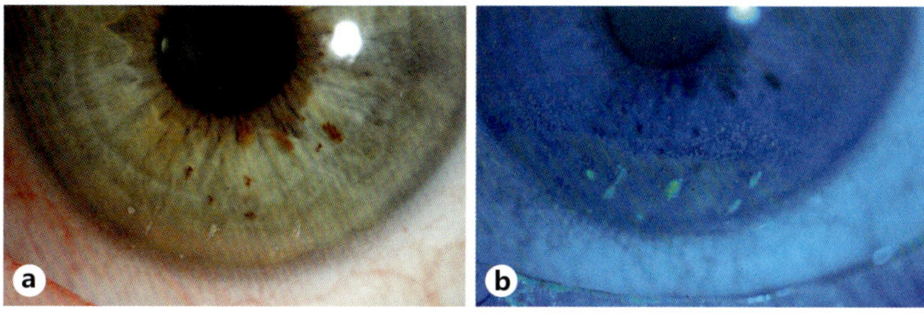

Fig. 7. a Filamentary keratitis in a patient with dry eye related to rheumatoid disease. Note the mucus accumulation around the filaments. **b** The same eye stained with fluorescein showing bright staining of the filaments and mucus blobs. Extensive superficial punctate keratitis is seen in the inferior cornea.

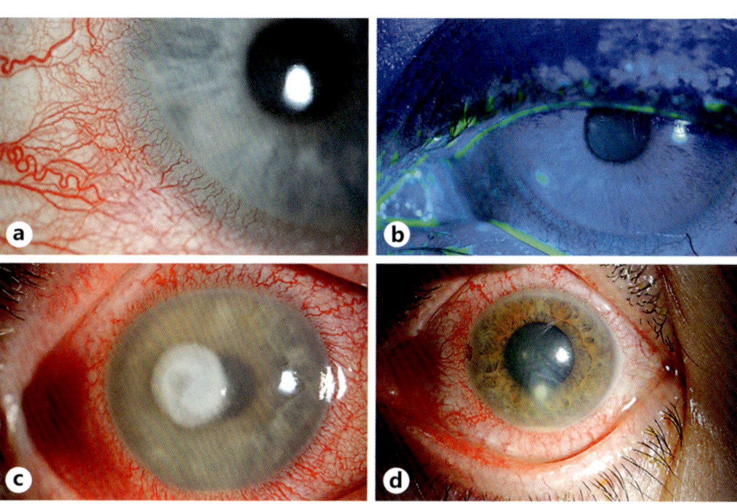

Fig. 8. a Peripheral corneal ulcer with infiltrates and an adjacent limbal injection. **b** Fluorescein staining shows a small ulcer. This ulcer would be regarded as not sight threatening. **c** Large central corneal ulcer more than 3 mm in diameter. **d** Central corneal ulcer in a contact lens wearer. The ulcer is small but is associated with considerable corneal oedema and hypopyon. Both (**c**) and (**d**) show sight-threatening ulcers.

Inflammation is recognized as an important player in the pathophysiology of dry eye. Drops of steroids and non-steroidal anti-inflammatory drugs (NSAIDs) are useful in combating inflammation at the outset of treatment, especially for moderate to severe dry eye. NSAIDs have the added advantage of analgesia, as well. In the long term, control of inflammation can be achieved with cyclosporin A (Restasis 0.05%), which spares the use of steroids [23]. Tacrolimus, like cyclosporin, is another specific calcineurin inhibitor that is available as an eye preparation in some countries or off-label as a skin cream (0.03%) that is applied to the eyes. Androgens and mucin stimulators are drugs that will be added to the dry eye pharmacopoeia in the near future [24]. Filaments (fig. 7a, b), when present, need to be individually picked out, as they tend to accumulate mucus and polymorphs and cause considerable irritation.

Infective Keratitis

Infective keratitis is often a very serious ocular emergency that requires prompt attention and management. Bacterial keratitis, the most common corneal infection worldwide, represents a significant cause of ocular morbidity. Low risk (non-sight-threatening) corneal infection, which is usually superficial, off-centre, and less than 3 mm in size (fig. 8a, b), with no history of contact lens wear, trauma, recurrent steroid use, immunosuppression or OS problems is usually empirically

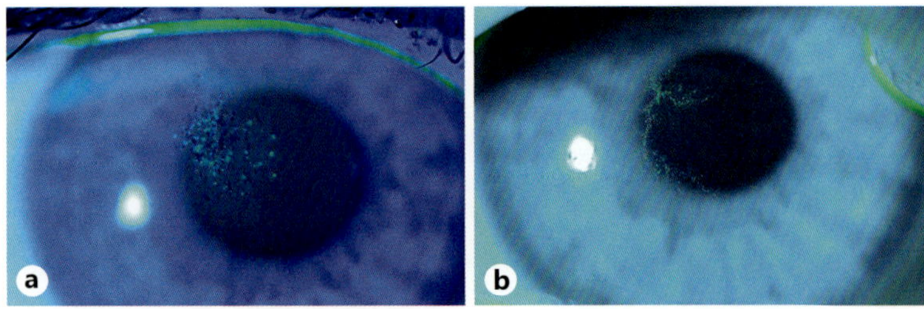

Fig. 9. a Epithelial manifestation of acanthamoeba keratitis in the form of coarse punctate keratitis in the central cornea. **b** The same patient presented 1 month later with an epithelial 'pseudodendrite' lesion (reproduced from author's publication [25]).

treated with topical fourth generation fluoroquinolones such as ciprofloxacin 0.3% or levofloxacin 0.5% hourly with close follow-up for response to treatment. Patients presenting with more severe (sight-threatening) infection (central or deep-seated and/or a large area of infection (fig. 8c, d) in the presence of signs of anterior chamber reaction, such as cells and flare) should have their lesions scraped from the base and sides of the ulcer, and samples of these lesions should be sent to the laboratory for direct smear examination and culture on various media (e.g. blood, chocolate, and non-nutrient agar). When acanthamoeba is suspected especially, with contact lens wear, and in cases of severe pain disproportionate to the signs, additional culture on non-nutrient agar (to prevent overgrowth of bacteria) enriched with *Escherichia coli* (on which the trophozoites feed and leave a characteristic trail) should be done. Samples should also be taken from the contact lens and cases. Occasionally, in early cases of acanthamoeba, there is no epithelial breakdown, and only minute subepithelial infiltrates (fig. 9a) are seen before the more characteristic pseudodendrites manifest (fig. 9b) [25]. In these cases, epithelial samples are collected from the area of the lesion together with scraping of the underlying tissue. Care should be taken not to break the surface of the agar when spreading the samples on the plate. Plating should be done in a 'C' pattern so that the observer is able to determine pathogen growth along the curve of the 'C' and to differentiate these from non-specific contaminants, which would grow randomly on the plate. The plates should be kept at room temperature for 20–30 minutes before plating to maximize results. When possible, an extra sample is put in broth to enhance organismal proliferation. Sabouraud agar is added when fungal infection is suspected, especially in endemic areas with a hot climate or in immunocompromised patients. Patients who are already on antibiotic drops at presentation should stop all medications 24–48 hours prior to sampling [26].

Once corneal scraping is performed, fortified antibiotics against both gram-positive and gram-negative bacteria should be started hourly around the clock for 48 hours (at our centre, we use Cefuroxime 10% and Gentamycin 1.5% eye drops prepared in our local pharmacy) in addition to cyclopentolate 1% (or atropine 1%) twice a day to reduce pain and ciliary spasm. An initial loading dose of each antibiotic instilled in an alternating manner every 5 minutes for half an hour can be useful. This regime can achieve corneal concentrations similar to that of subconjunctival injection. Response to treatment is assessed daily. If clinical improvement is seen, treatment is continued even if the sensitivity from the culture result is different, with gradual tapering of the drops to 2 per hour and further tapering that is tailored to the case (fig. 10). In no case should antibiotics be tapered to a dose below their minimum inhibitory concentration (instillation of the usual concentration approximately four times a day). If there is no response or if the response is inadequate, consider changing antibiotics guided by the culture results. Amikacin 0.2% eye drops (or fortified 2.5–3%) prepared from vials for

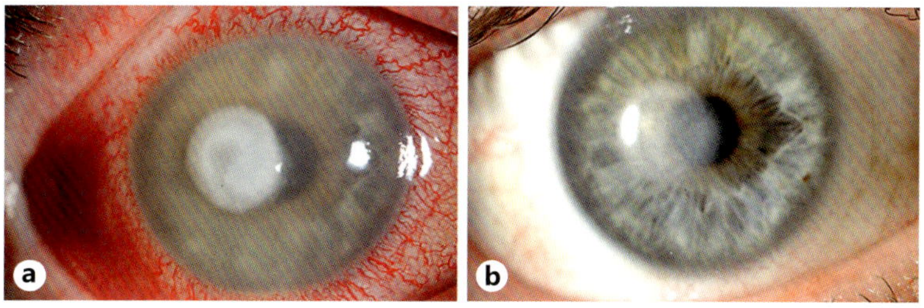

Fig. 10. a Active corneal ulcer treated with fortified antibiotics (cefuroxime 10% and gentamicin 1.5%) hourly for 24 hours and then tapered in accordance with the clinical response. **b** After complete healing. A macular grade scar is left. In such cases, a rigid gas-permeable contact lens should be tried before contemplating keratoplasty.

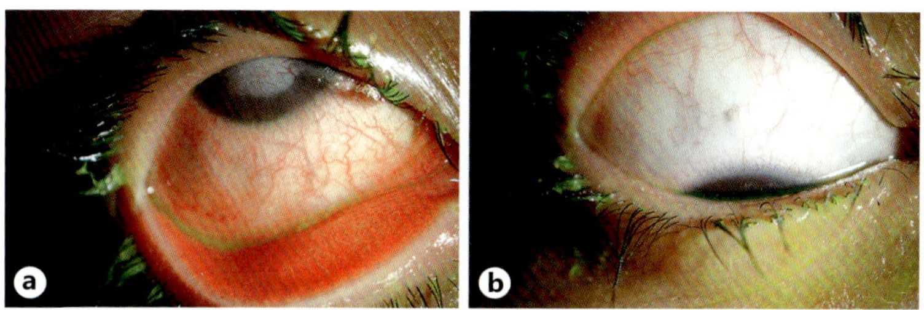

Fig. 11. The 'up-down sign' of drug toxicity at the ocular surface. When the patient looks up (**a**), the lower bulbar and forniceal conjunctiva show intense congestion. The inferior bulbar conjunctiva may also show epithelial defects when stained with fluorescein. When the patient looks down (**b**), the upper bulbar and forniceal conjunctiva are white. (Reproduced from author's publication [27].)

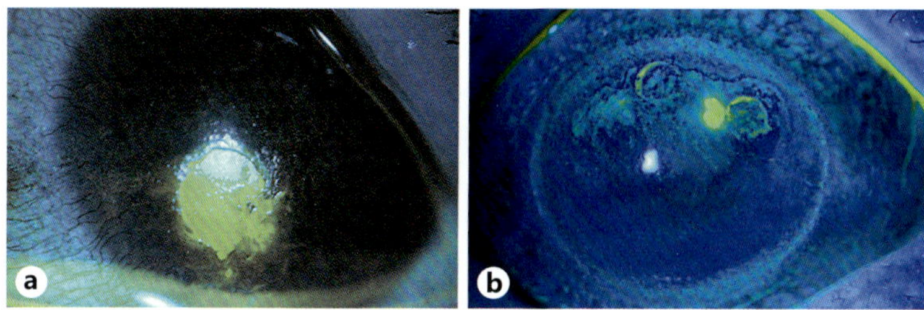

Fig. 12. a Epithelial biopsy. When the pathology is primarily epithelial, the inflammation and oedema make the epithelium loose, and it can easily be peeled off the surface of the cornea. **b** Stromal biopsy of sites overlapping the lesion with a 3 mm skin biopsy punch. One sample was processed for microbiology, and the other sample was processed for histopathology.

parenteral use is effective for gram-negative infections such as Pseudomonas, although this can be quite toxic to the cornea. Epithelial toxicity can retard epithelial healing and increase patient discomfort and intolerance. Drug toxicity can be identified by asking the patient to look down and up to observe the bulbar conjunctiva. A marked increase in redness and injection in the lower half compared to the upper half, the 'up-down sign' (fig. 11a, b), is representative of drug toxicity [27] and is an indication to taper, change or reduce the strength of the preparation (e.g. change from gentamycin 1.5% fortified antibiotic to commercially available 0.3%).

If no response is seen with conventional therapy, all medications should be stopped for 48 hours, and the scrape should be repeated or multiple corneal biopsies should be taken from the (advancing) edge of the lesion with adjacent normal tissue. A sheet of loose epithelium can be peeled off intact (fig. 12a). Alternatively, biopsies can be done with skin biopsy punches of 2 or 3 mm in diameter and be processed for microbial and histological evaluation (fig. 12b).

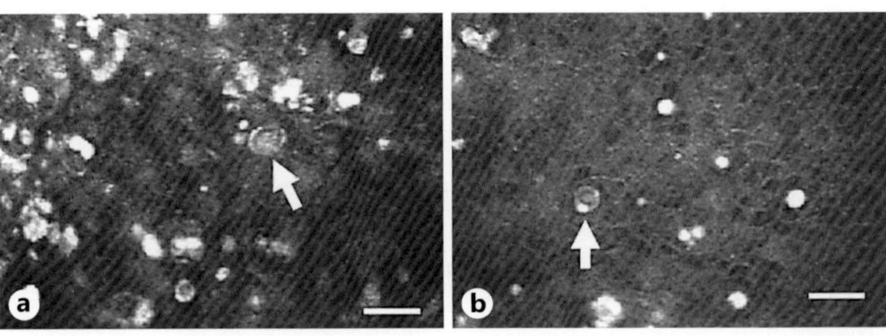

Fig. 13. In vivo confocal images of acanthamoeba cysts showing the bright spot and double-walled (arrow) appearance in (**a**) and a signet ring appearance in (**b**, arrow). (Reproduced from author's publication [25].)

In patients presenting with a high index of suspicion for acanthamoeba infection (history of contact lens wear, subepithelial infiltrate, limbitis, radial keratoneuritis and ring or double ring infiltrates), in vivo confocal microscopy can be done to visualize acanthamoeba cysts, which appear as bright hyper-reflective lesions, double-walled or signet ring cysts (fig. 13a, b). Though not conclusive, the presence of many clusters of cysts in different sites, especially in the stroma, is highly suggestive [28]. Sometimes, acanthamoeba infection manifests as (pseudo)dendritiform epithelial lesions, which could be mistaken for herpes simplex keratitis. Similarly, associated anterior chamber reaction can mislead one to diagnose and treat the disease as iritis with topical steroids, which can lead to disease progression. Culture results may take up to 3 weeks, and the results are only positive in 50% of clinically suspected cases. Many studies have shown that early treatment, within 3 weeks, is associated with better visual prognosis [29].

Treatment is usually started with a combination of Biguanide (Polyhexamethyline bigunides 0.02% or Chlorhexidine 0.02%), which is effective against the cyst form, and Diamidine (Propamidine 0.1% or Hexamidine 0.1%), which is effective against both the cyst and trophozoite forms. Drops are administered every hour around the clock for 48 hours initially, followed by hourly day-only drops, and these treatments are tapered gradually according to the response [26].

Steroid use is controversial. However, it can be used to control a persistent OS and anterior chamber inflammatory reaction after adequate response to anti-acanthamoebic therapy is seen. Anti-acanthamoebic therapy should be continued for 4 weeks after steroid withdrawal to abort any active infection from viable cysts. Associated limbitis and scleritis can usually be controlled with oral NSAIDS or oral cyclosporine, with anti-amoebic cover such as oral itraconazole 100 mg/day to prevent spread to adjacent tissue [30]. In keratitis cases in which the initial response to antibacterial agents is followed by cessation of the treatment response or worsening of the condition, co-infection with bacteria and acanthamoeba and/or fungus should be suspected. Oral tetracycline, as an antiprotease agent, helps to limit stromal melts and should be considered in all cases of infective keratitis in which the risk of corneal melting is high.

Viral Infections
Herpes simplex virus type 1 is the most common cause of viral infection of the OS. It can affect many parts of the ocular tissue, such as the lids, the conjunctiva, the cornea, the uvea and the retina. Following primary infection, which can present as conjunctivitis, vesicles and ulcers on the lids or even corneal dendritic ulcers, the virus remains latent in the trigeminal ganglia. Viral reactivation can lead to recurrent infection in the form of epithelial, stromal or endothelial disease. Patients presenting with epithelial keratitis often have pain, redness, photophobia and blurred vision. A dendritic ulcer can be visualized by fluorescein staining and can progress to a geographic ulcer

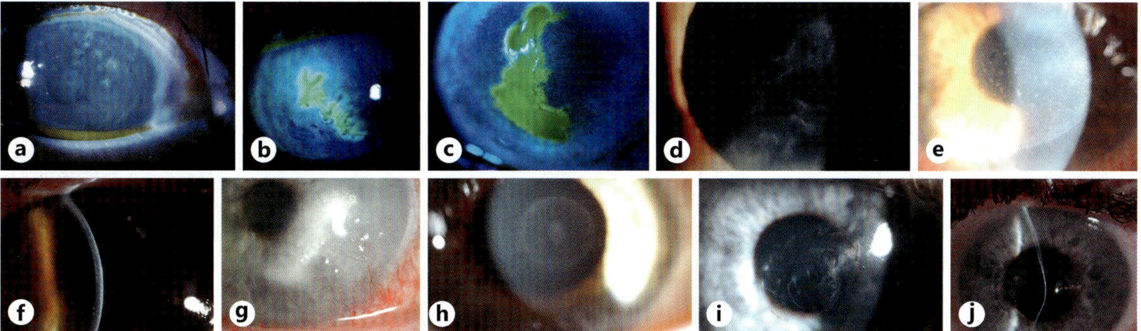

Fig. 14. Corneal epithelial manifestation of herpes simplex infection. **a** Microdendrites. **b** Dendritic ulcer. **c** Geographic ulcer. **a–c** show eyes stained with fluorescein. These lesions represent active viral replication. **d** Ghost dendrite, which is seen at times after the healing of a dendritic/geographic lesion. **e** Stromal disciform keratitis. At the defined edge of the lesion, keratic precipitates and epithelial vesicles due to oedema are clearly seen. **f** Slit image of the same eye as presented in (**e**) showing stromal oedema. **g** Interstitial keratitis manifesting as stromal infiltration with superficial and deep vessels. **h** A clearly defined immune ring (Wessley's ring) on the cornea. This represents immune complex precipitation in the corneal stroma. **i** Extreme corneal thinning and ectasia following chronic herpetic keratitis. **j** The thinning is very evident on the slit image.

spontaneously or if improperly treated with topical steroids (fig. 14a–d). Epithelial disease is caused by direct viral replication and cytopathic effects. Treatment with Acyclovir ointment 3% used 5 times/day for 1–2 weeks is usually effective. In resistant cases, Gancyclovir gel 0.15% can be used 3 times/day. Other antiviral drugs such as trifluorothymidine, Vira A and Famvir can also be effective [31].

Herpetic stromal keratitis (fig. 14e–h) predominantly results from an immune-mediated reaction to the viral proteins and leads to corneal-localized oedema surrounded by an immune ring (Wessely ring, fig. 14h) or generalized oedema with eventual vascularization and opacity (fig. 14e–g). The severe form of necrotizing stromal keratitis with corneal melting is rare and requires aggressive treatment. Stromal keratitis can lead to extreme thinning and ectasia of the cornea (fig. 14i, j). Herpetic stromal keratitis is treated with frequent administration of topical steroids under the cover of systemic antiviral agents. Recurrence is a hallmark of viral infections. Patients with frequent recurrence (more than twice/year) should be maintained on long-term antiviral cover. Recurrent herpetic keratitis may lead to reduced corneal sensation and neurotropic keratitis, which is often resistant to treatment by lubricants and which requires surgical intervention, such as tarsorrhaphy or the temporary induction of ptosis by botulinum toxin (Botox), to protect the OS [32]. Herpes zoster infection can affect the OS in the form of lid erythema, conjunctivitis and dendritic ulcers, which are often self-limiting but can lead to neurotrophic keratitis in up to 25% of cases [33]. Other viral infections such as adenovirus can cause self-limiting keratoconjunctivitis, which may not need treatment other than symptomatic relief by topical steroids in severe cases.

Fungal Keratitis
Corneal fungal infection presents a challenge to ophthalmologists all over the world with respect to both diagnosis and treatment. Often, ophthalmologists have to start antifungal treatment based on clinical suspicion. Direct smear seen with potassium hydroxide wet mount or haematoxylin and eosin stain may show fungal hyphae or spores, which could give guidance in initiating treatment. The culture results may take up to

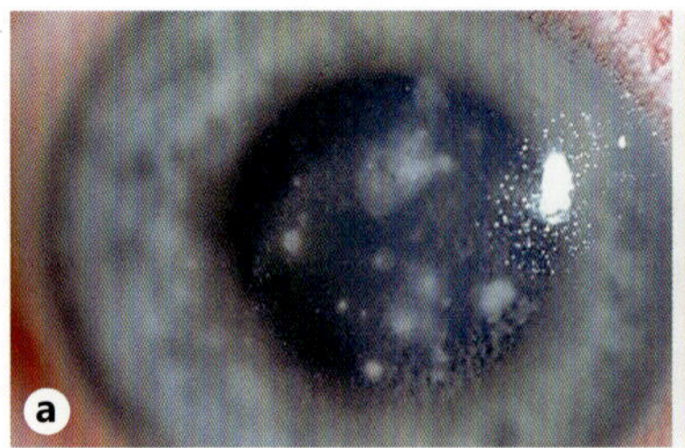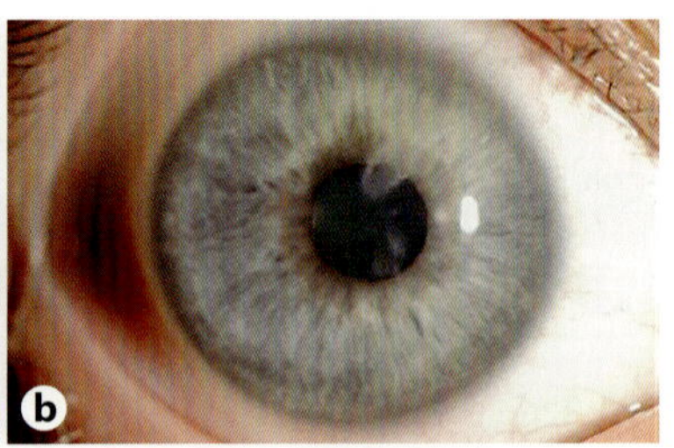

Fig. 15. Fungal keratitis. **a** Active Candida infection post-laser in situ keratomileusis showing multiple foci of infection. **b** After successful treatment with Amphotericin eye drops.

3 weeks. Although polymerase chain reaction of corneal scrape samples can produce reliable results in 24–48 hours, this assay is very expensive and is not readily available at most centres [34].

Broad-spectrum antifungal agents are not available even as off-label preparations. First line treatment can include a combination of hourly drops of Econazole 1% (which is more effective against filamentous fungi such as Aspergillus and Fusarium spp.) and Amphoterycin B 0.1–0.3% (which is the drug of choice for Candida and other related yeast infections). The drops could be tapered gradually according to the response. Alternatively, Natamycin, which is the only commercially available topical antifungal drop preparation, can be used for superficial infections, as it has low penetration into the cornea and a limited therapeutic spectrum.

Other antifungal agents such as azoles (ketoconazole, miconazole, fluconazole, itraconazole, econazole, and clotrimazole) can be reconstituted and used as eye drops or systemically with a broad-spectrum therapeutic effect. Upon systemic administration, they reach a good concentration in the anterior chamber and can be used for deep-seated infections. Fluconazole has better corneal penetration than other azoles and may be associated with fewer adverse effects. Echinocandins, such as Micafungin, Caspofungin and Anidulafungin, were shown to be fungicidal against various Candida species while fungistatic against Aspergillus species. New generation triazoles, including Voriconazole, Posaconazole and Ravuconazole, have been shown to have an excellent susceptibil-

ity profile and fewer side effects. Fluorinated pyrimidines such as Flucytosine have a synergistic effect if administered with azoles or Amphotericin B but on their own may lead to the emergence of resistant strains. Antiseptics such as Chlorhexidine 0.2% and Povidone iodine (5%) have also been advocated as cheap and readily available alternatives or adjuvants (for microbial keratitis) but may not be as effective on their own as other specific agents. Often, one may resort to combined routes of administration of antifungal agents in cases of severe keratitis or keratoscleritis. Subconjunctival injections every 12 hours can sometimes be effective when the response to topical drops is slow or inadequate. Repeated intracameral injection of antifungal agents (e.g. Amphotericin B, 5 mg in 0.1 ml of 5% dextrose) has been tried to treat deep-seated infections [35]. Intrastromal injection of Voriconazole (50 mg in 0.1 ml) at the junction of the infiltrate and the healthy corneal tissue in deep-seated filamentous keratitis cases has been tried with promising results [36]. Steroid use in fungal keratitis is controversial and must be deferred until a definitive therapeutic response is seen (fig. 15a, b).

Intraocular pressure can be normal, high or low in eyes with microbial keratitis. In the presence of a corneal ulcer or abscess, the use of a Goldman tonometer may not be ideal. The Tonopen is better suited for pressure measurement, and disposable caps are more suited for the prevention of contamination of the instrument tip. Often, digital assessment (finger palpation) may be the only suitable way to assess pressure, depending on the clinician's experience. It is

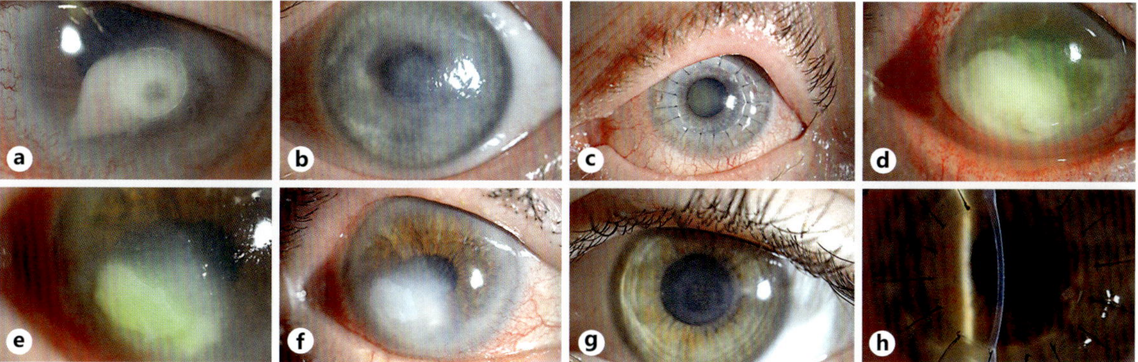

Fig. 16. Surgical management of microbial keratitis. **a** Corneal perforation in Candida keratitis sealed with cyanoacrylate glue. **b, c** Active chronic infective keratitis (mixed bacterial and acanthamoeba) treated with a therapeutic graft. Cataract surgery was not done at the same time to avoid the risk of capsular bag/vitreous contamination. **d** Severe microbial keratitis non-responsive to fortified antibiotics. **e** The lesion responded when an amniotic membrane patch was glued to the surface of the ulcer/abscess. **f** Complete healing of the lesion with an amniotic membrane graft in situ. **g, h** Post-infectious keratitis central scar treated with deep anterior lamellar keratoplasty.

important that the pressure be assessed often during the course of an infection and that the infection be appropriately treated if required (oral acetazolamide may be more convenient than topical antiglaucoma medications).

Surgical Options for Infective Keratitis

Corneal Gluing. In severe cases with stromal melting and descemetocele or frank perforation, corneal gluing is a useful option. Perforations of 3 mm or less are better suited for closure with glue. Both cyanoacrylate glue and fibrin glue have been used to good effect. With cyanoacrylate glue, a bandage contact lens is required to cover the rough surface of the glue, as eyelid contact during blinks can be damaging to the lids and can cause the glue to become displaced (fig. 16a).

Therapeutic Grafts. When larger perforations occur, therapeutic keratoplasty may be the only option to control the infection and re-form the globe. Therapeutic grafts are not without complications, such as recurrence of infection, intractable glaucoma and rejection, and should be used as a last resort [37] (fig. 16b, c).

Paracentesis. Paracentesis in the presence of active infection is controversial and should be avoided whenever possible. Any hypopyon (except fungal) is usually sterile, and paracentesis should not be performed for culture of organisms as the risk of intraocular spread of infection is high. Occasionally, this procedure is carried out to reduce eye pressure when other measures have failed.

Amniotic Membrane and Conjunctival Flaps. In intractable infections, either gluing or suturing AM to the affected area has been shown to induce a favourable response to ongoing treatment. The exact mechanism of action of AM is unknown, but it is believed that the AM acts as a reservoir of the instilled medication and concentrates drug delivery to the site of infection [38, 39] (fig. 16d–f).

Conjunctival hooding, or the Gunderson flap, can be a good option to help the vascularization and healing of severe infective keratitis. Collagen cross-linking can be employed to good effect in refractive cases, as well. Studies have shown that corneal crosslinking helps in controlling the infection and preventing melting in severe infectious keratitis cases [40].

Keratoplasty. Stromal scars resulting from infective keratitis can be nebular, macular or

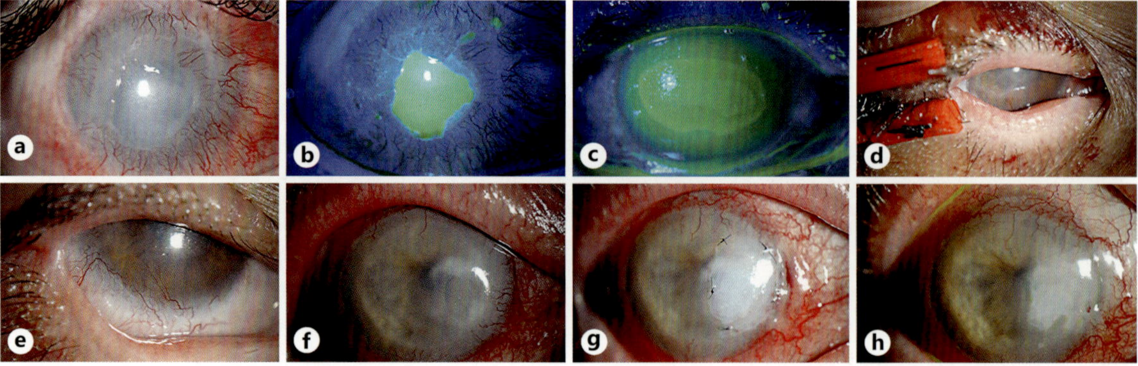

Fig. 17. a, b Persistent epithelial defect following a chemical burn. **c** A persistent neurotrophic ulcer following herpes zoster ophthalmicus. **d, e** Persistent epithelial defect treated with a permanent lateral tarsorrhaphy. The ulcer remained healed after the rubber bolsters were removed. **f–h** A persistent epithelial defect following bacterial keratitis was treated with a multi-layered amniotic membrane graft. The sutures were removed after the amniotic membrane was covered by corneal epithelium.

leucoma (adherent leukoma) grade. They can cause irregular astigmatism and visual impairment even when not directly in the visual axis. When in the visual axis, they interfere with the entrance of light into the eye and reduce vision. A trial of a rigid gas-permeable contact lens should be given before contemplating corneal transplantation. Often, reasonable visual improvement can be gained with rigid gas-permeable lenses. When corneal transplantation is required, deep anterior lamellar keratoplasty is the procedure of choice, but in cases of deep melts, descemetocoeles and perforations, a penetrating keratoplasty may be the better option (fig. 16g, h).

Persistent Corneal Epithelial Defects

A persistent corneal epithelial defect is one that does not heal or that heals and breaks down repeatedly. It can be associated with stromal (substrate) pathology or can be secondary to infections or immune-mediated keratopathy, leading to the following: perforation; poor corneal sensation (neurotrophic) secondary to nerve damage, which can be iatrogenic, or secondary to trauma,

infection (herpes simplex and zoster) or tumours; problems with epithelial regeneration (LSCD); exposure (facial palsy) and systemic associations such as diabetes mellitus, vitamin A and other nutritional deficiencies (fig. 17a–c).

Medical Management
A variety of agents can be used individually or in combination. These agents include topical lubricants – preservative-free drops, gels and ointments, sodium hyaluronate, autologous serum (20–100%) and autologous plasma. Fibronectin and epidermal growth factor alone or together have been shown to be beneficial but are not popular. The use of nerve growth factor and substance P peptide hold considerable promise but are not widely available yet. Cacicol, a structural analogue of glycosaminoglycan, is relatively new and is described as a regenerating agent. It contains the polymer, polycarboxymethylglucose sulphate, which is an analogue of the extracellular matrix glycosaminoglycan heparan sulphate. When topically administered, it replaces degraded heparan sulphate and interacts with structural proteins and growth factors to promote healing. It also helps protect matrix proteins from

degradation by increasing their resistance to gly-canases (enzymes).

Other measures such as a patch and a bandage to firmly close the eyelids or a bandage contact lens can be used together with medical measures. Several surgical options for the treatment of persistent corneal epithelial defects are available and should be tailored to the underlying condition. The available treatment options comprise temporary or (semi) permanent lid closure via botulinum injection, tarsorrhaphy (gold standard) (fig. 17d, e), an AM patch or graft (overlay or inlay) (fig. 17f–h), conjunctival grafts (free grafts or flaps) and limbal SC transplantation (explants or ex vivo expanded sheets). Both AM and conjunctival grafts can be attached in place with fibrin glue. When there is associated tear deficiency, punctal plugs or punctal cautery can be useful [32].

Allergic Eye Disease

Allergic reactions are classically categorized into four different types:

Type 1: immediate hypersensitivity, e.g. hay fever;

Type 2: antibody-mediated hypersensitivity reactions, such as blood transfusion reactions;

Type 3: immune complex-mediated disease, including serum sickness and some auto-immune diseases (e.g. systemic lupus erythematosus); and

Type 4: delayed hypersensitivity, e.g. contact dermatitis and contact conjunctivitis, or allograft rejection.

Allergic diseases affecting the OS are of six main types:
- acute allergic conjunctivitis,
- seasonal allergic conjunctivitis (SAC),
- perennial allergic conjunctivitis,
- vernal keratoconjunctivitis (VKC),
- atopic keratoconjunctivitis (AKC), and
- giant papillary conjunctivitis.

Acute allergic conjunctivitis is a type 1 (immediate hypersensitivity) disease which occurs at any age, especially in childhood. It affects atopes and non-atopes with symptoms of intense itching and swelling of the conjunctiva (chemosis) and the eyelids. It is self-limiting and normally requires no treatment. Atopy is the body's ability to mount a specific IgE response upon exposure to an allergen. When excessive, the individual is said to be atopic. Approximately half of atopic individuals suffer from allergic disease.

SAC is also an immediate hypersensitivity reaction to pollens, which manifests as the ocular component of hay fever; history generally points to the diagnosis. Watering, itching, redness and mucoid discharge are usual symptoms affecting both eyes. Chemosis and lid swelling are usually present, but the cornea is not involved.

Perennial allergic conjunctivitis, as the name suggests, has a year-round incidence and is another immediate hypersensitivity reaction. The clinical manifestations resemble SAC, but the condition is much rarer. Dust mite is a common causative allergen, but other allergens that are present throughout the year can also be responsible (fig. 18a).

VKC has a complex pathogenesis involving all types of hypersensitivity reactions. It has a geographical and racial variation and can lead to visual impairment secondary to corneal involvement. Microbial infections may co-exist. Micro- and macropapillae affecting the conjunctiva are a classic clinical sign. Corneal erosions, subepithelial scarring and plaques, limbal inflammation and Taranta's dots are other important signs (fig. 18b, c).

AKC is a disease that is observed in atopic adults who have eczema of facial and eyelid skin. Like VKC, it has a complex pathogenesis and affects the cornea and threatens sight. Other ocular associations include keratoconus, cataract and retinal detachment.

Giant papillary conjunctivitis is characterized by giant (>1 mm) papillae, usually in the upper tarsal conjunctiva, limbal inflammation, hyperaemia and oedema, but this disease does not involve the cornea [41] (fig. 18d).

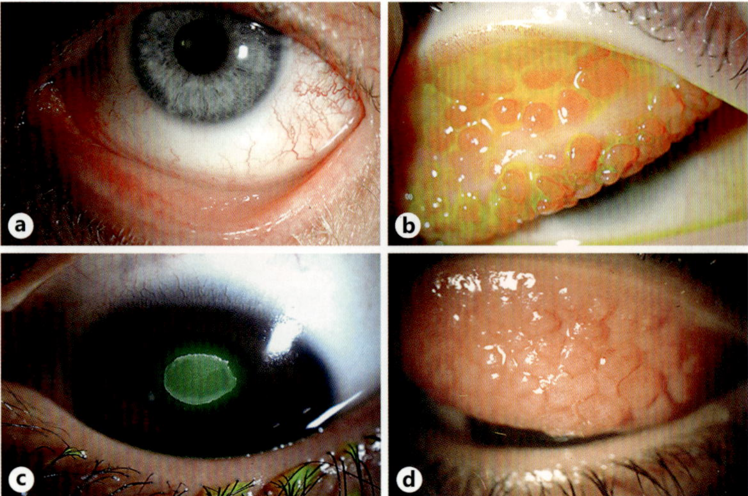

Fig. 18. a Conjunctival, especially palpebral, congestion in seasonal allergic conjunctivitis. **b** Large papillae in vernal keratoconjunctivitis. **c** Vernal plaque on the cornea. **d** Giant papillary conjunctivitis.

Management

The drugs used in the treatment of OS allergic disease include the following (some trade names are given in parentheses):

Antihistamines (H1): Emedastine difumarate (Emadine), Levocabastine, Epinastine (Elestat), and Azelastine ophthalmic (Optivar);

Mast cell stabilizers (also H1): Lodoxamide tromethamine (Alomide), Olopatadine (Patanol), Ketotifen (Zaditor), Neodocromil, and Cromoglycate (opticrom);

NSAIDS: Ketorolac tromethamine (Acular), and Diclofenac (Voltarol);

Steroids: Dexamethasone, Betamethasone, Prednisolone acetate, Fluromethalone, Remixilone, and Loteprednol;

Immunosuppressive agents: Cyclosporine 0.05–2%) and Protopic (tacrolimus) skin cream, 0.03%; and

Artificial tears and mucolytics: Acetylcystine (Ilube), which acts as a mucolytic agent.

The excision of plaques and, rarely giant papillae, cryotherapy for giant papillae, superficial keratectomy, and the injection of steroids into the tarsal conjunctiva are minor surgical interventions that may be required.

Symptoms of itching and swelling respond to antihistamines and mast cell stabilisers. The latter can also be used for prophylaxis during the pollen season. NSAIDs help to reduce inflammation. In more severe cases, especially AKC, steroids and NSAIDs are required. In AKC with eczema and asthma, systemic cyclosporine can help manage both eye and skin manifestations. Systemic medication such as antihistamines may also be required when non-ocular manifestations are present (hay fever) (table 1).

Ocular Cicatricial Pemphigoid

Ocular cicatricial pemphigoid (OCP) is a progressive cicatrizing condition of the skin and mucosal surfaces, especially the eye and oral mucosa [42]. It is bilateral with a chronic course of remittance and relapse associated with acute exacerbations. Its exact cause is unknown, but it is known to occur after viral, bacterial or other infections and is associated with systemic (beta blockers, e.g. Practalol) and topical antiglaucoma medication use.

Its pathogenesis is related to the deposition of complement-fixing antibodies against the

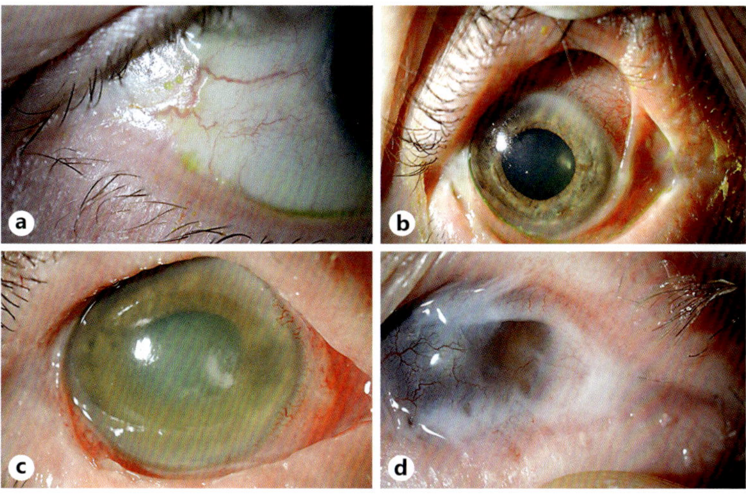

Fig. 19. Ocular cicatricial pemphigoid. **a** Scarring of canthal conjunctiva with keratinization. Note how the drops instilled in the conjunctival sac stay as globules on the surface of the keratin. **b** Conjunctival scarring (symblepharon) in OCP. The cornea remains uninvolved. **c** Corneal involvement with infiltration, haziness and limbal vascularization in OCP. **d** End-stage OCP.

Table 1. Summary table for allergic eye disease

Disease	Age group	Cornea involved	Morbidity	Need for steroids
AAC	Any (especially infants)	No	Low	Zero
SAC	10–40 years, peak 20–30 years	No	Low to moderate	Zero
PAC	Similar to SAC	No	Low to moderate	Zero to low
VKC	Onset: 82% <10 years	Yes	High	High
AKC	Young adults	Yes	High	High
GPC	CL wearers, etc.	No	Moderate	Zero to low

AAC = Acute allergic conjunctivitis; CL = contact lens; GPC = giant papillary conjunctivitis; PAC = perennial allergic conjunctivitis.

conjunctival basement membrane proteins laminin and integrin (Type II reaction). This attracts lymphocytes, macrophages and neutrophils, which release enzymes and growth factors. The proteolytic and collagenolytic enzymes cause tissue damage, and the growth factors stimulate fibroblast proliferation and induce scarring.

Clinical Features

Females are more affected than males at a ratio of 2:1 among those over 60 years of age. Subepithelial bullae appear and are replaced by cicatrizing connective tissue, resulting in mucosal shrinkage. The buccal mucosa is involved in 85% of cases, and the skin in 25%. The onset is asymmetrical, manifesting in one eye before the other. In the early stages, repeated episodes of mild to moderate conjunctival inflammation and vascular injection occur. Other signs of papillae, chemosis, ulcerations and vesicles may also be present [42]. Classically, its progression is divided into 4 stages (fig. 19a–d):

Stage 1: conjunctival inflammation, mucoid discharge, rose Bengal staining of the conjunctiva, and subtle conjunctival subepithelial fibrosis;

Stage 2: conjunctival shrinkage, most notably in the inferior fornix;

Stage 3: advanced shrinkage, symblephara, keratopathy, corneal vascularization, trichiasis and tear film abnormalities; and

Stage 4: end-stage disease, severe keratoconjunctivitis sicca, keratinization, and ankyloblepharon.

Dry eye is a feature that is secondary to the following: the loss of goblet cells causing mucin deficiency; cicatrization of the lacrimal gland ducts, causing aqueous deficiency; and scarring and keratinization of the meibomian glands, causing lipid deficiency. Persistent severe dryness leads to keratinization of the conjunctiva and the cornea.

Treatment of Ocular Cicatricial Pemphigoid

The primary goals of therapy are to suppress inflammation and to inhibit the progression of conjunctival shrinkage. Other therapeutic goals include the replacement of the tear film, the restoration of the normal eyelid-OS anatomic relationship and the maintenance or re-establishment of a clear central cornea. Aggressive lubrication and timely and swift management of episodes of infection (manifesting as discharge and red sticky eyes) with topical antibiotics is required.

Dapsone (diaminodiphenylsulfone) is often used as the first line drug for patients with early-stage OCP starting at 50 mg TID for 2 weeks and then decreasing to 50 mg OD depending on the response. Full blood counts need to be monitored very closely. The drug should be avoided in patients with glucose-6-phosphate dehydrogenase deficiency or sulfa allergy. Haemolytic anaemia and methaemoglobinaemia can occur as adverse events.

Cyclophosphamide, the drug of choice for severe and progressive disease, can be given orally or as intravenous pulse therapy. Other immunosuppressant agents such as azathioprine and mycophenolate have also proved beneficial. These are used either together with steroids (oral or pulsed intravenous) or after remission has been induced by steroids. Co-management with a physician (immunologist/rheumatologist) is a standard approach [43].

Surgical Management
Surgery should generally be avoided, as trauma leads to a worsening of symptoms and signs. When required, surgery should be undertaken when the eye is quiet. Introduction of immunosuppression with steroids or other agents should be considered in the perioperative period.

Surgical options include punctal occlusion for severe dry eyes and epilation, electrolysis or lash excision for trichiasis. This can be complemented by the use of mini scleral lenses (Boston lens) to protect the cornea. Lid malpositioning may require surgical correction especially to prevent trauma to the OS caused by altered lid margins and/or eyelashes. AM grafting may help with the release of adhesions or symblephara or to aid OS re-epithelialization in the presence of persistent epithelial defects.

Limbal SC transplants (in vivo or ex vivo) and penetrating keratoplasty are needed in the later stages for visual rehabilitation but should be undertaken only when the disease is inactive, the eye is moist, and there are no eyelid abnormalities. These grafts are at high risk of rejection [44]. Prosthokeratoplasty is the only hope for visual rehabilitation in many of these patients with end-stage disease.

Erythema Multiforme Major (Stevens-Johnson Syndrome)

Stevens-Johnson syndrome (SJS) is an acute blistering disease involving the skin and the mucous membrane with occasional recurrent ocular inflammation in which corneal damage is one of the most common long-term sequelae. Eighty percent of patients who require hospitalization will develop OS sequelae, which are severe in up to 25% of patients [45].

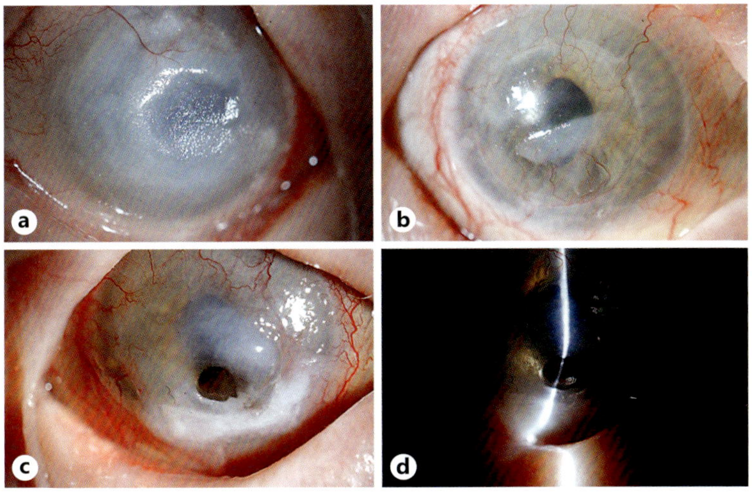

Fig. 20. Stevens-Johnson syndrome (SJS). **a** Severe dry eye with complete keratinisation of the cornea in SJS. **b** A failing corneal graft in SJS with superficial and deep vascularization. **c** Deep stromal melt with extensive scarring in SJS. **d** Slit beam image of the eye presented in (**c**) showing corneal melt down to Descemet's membrane.

SJS is considered as a severe cutaneous adverse effect that is predominantly secondary to a drug reaction but that can also be induced by infection. Withdrawal of the implicated drug and treatment of the infection may affect the prognosis of this disease. It can be induced by a variety of drugs, of which the most common are antibiotics (such as penicillin, sulfonamides, cephalosporins, quinolones and antimalarials) and anti-inflammatory drugs (such as ibuprofen and mephanamic acid). Other drugs such as antiepileptic medications (phenytoin and carbamazepines), salbutamol and promethazine have also been implicated [46]. SJS is believed to be a T cell-mediated reaction specifically involving CD8 lymphocytes and natural killer cells, which are identified as the most important factors in epidermal destruction [47].

After the acute episode, symptoms and signs can vary from mild to severe forms of conjunctival inflammation with or without progressive cicatrization and later keratinization of OS structures including the lids, the conjunctiva, and the meibomian orifices and lacrimal ducts, which can result in severe dry eye (fig. 20a–d). Recurrent trauma to the OS due to blinking can precipitate intractable ulceration and corneal opacification, vascularization and scarring.

Limbal SC failure can set in after the acute episode or after many years of recurrent inflammation, resembling mucous membrane pemphigoid. In these cases, linear IgG deposits on immunofluorescence staining of conjunctival biopsy samples can be found in up to 50% of cases; thus, a good positive result confirms disease, but a negative result cannot rule out the diagnosis. Recurrent scleritis is another rare complication that can set in after the acute episode and can lead to a severe form of necrotizing scleritis [48].

In the acute stage of the disease, while patients are hospitalized with OS ulcerations and inflammation, it is helpful to use an AM. We have used an AM wrapped around a conformer and inserted it into the conjunctival sac under topical anaesthesia to improve patient comfort and to reduce the adhesions between the lid and the globe (fig. 21). 'ProKera', a commercially available AM with a conformer ring, though much more expensive, has been used with reported success to heal the corneal and conjunctival ulceration with limited adhesions and excellent visual acuity and outcomes [49].

The management of the chronic ocular sequelae of SJS is often tedious and challenging. It involves protecting and supporting the OS with

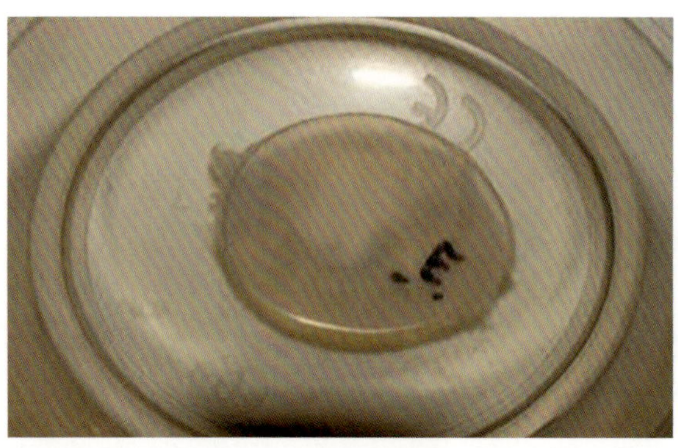

Fig. 21. An eye shield is wrapped with amniotic membrane for use to cover the globe and maintain the fornices. This can be used in patients with SJS and chemical burns.

tear substitutes, autologous serum, punctal plugs or cautery and aggressive control of the recurrent inflammation whilst minimizing drug toxicity.

External triggering factors of OS inflammation such as trichiasis and dystichiasis should be addressed so as not to mask the endogenous inflammation triggered by SJS [50]. However, any surgery to correct lid deformities such as entropion and exposure involving conjunctival manipulation or cataract surgery should be deferred until the disease is controlled with systemic immunosuppression [51]. Residual endogenous inflammation should be treated aggressively with systemic immunosuppression such as steroids, cyclosporine and other steroid-sparing agents. Sulfonamides are contraindicated, as they may aggravate or precipitate recurrence [52]. Reports have shown that the use of a high dose of cyclosporine and intravenous immunoglobulins early in the acute stage hold promise for reducing the mortality and long-term sequelae of SJS [53]. Topical steroids are often inadequate for the long-term control of ocular inflammation in SJS [54].

The management of LSCD should be deferred until at least 18 months after stabilization of the disease. Because of bilateral affection, visual rehabilitation is limited to allolimbal SC transplantation with a guarded prognosis and osteo-odonto-keratoprosthesis, which may be the only resort in cases with severe dry OS.

Limbal Stem Cell Deficiency and Limbal Transplant Surgery

Corneal epithelial SCs reside in the palisades of Vogt at the limbus. These cells sustain the entire corneal epithelial cell mass over the duration of the life of the individual. The evidence for the limbal location of corneal epithelial SCs is derived from clinical studies on corneal epithelial wound healing, histology including immunohistology and molecular biology.

Corneal epithelial wounds can be of three different types: (1) with an intact limbus, (2) with partial involvement of the limbus and (3) with total limbus involvement. In the first type, healing of the epithelial defect usually occurs with complete restoration of the corneal phenotype of the cells. Centripetal migration of cells occurs from the limbus in the form of 3–6 convex-fronted sheets. In the second type, the limbus can be repopulated either by cells from the remaining intact limbus by a preferential circumferential migration of cells along the denuded limbus, restoring limbal integrity for healing to proceed as in type one, or by the encroachment of conjunctival cells onto the cornea across the limbal defect. The latter pattern leads to partial LSCD. In type 3, the corneal surface can only be covered by conjunctiva-derived epithelium, usually resulting in total LSCD [12, 55].

A number of conditions can lead to LSCD. Aniridia, chemical burns, prolonged contact lens wear and chronic inflammatory conditions such as OCP and SJS are examples. LSCD can result in a number of pathological changes ranging from metaplastic epithelium on the cornea to complete corneal breakdown (fig. 22a–d). The diagnosis of LSCD is essentially clinical, and the demonstration of goblet cells in the corneal epithelium by impression cytology or biopsy can be confirmatory. The extent of LSCD is usually classed as

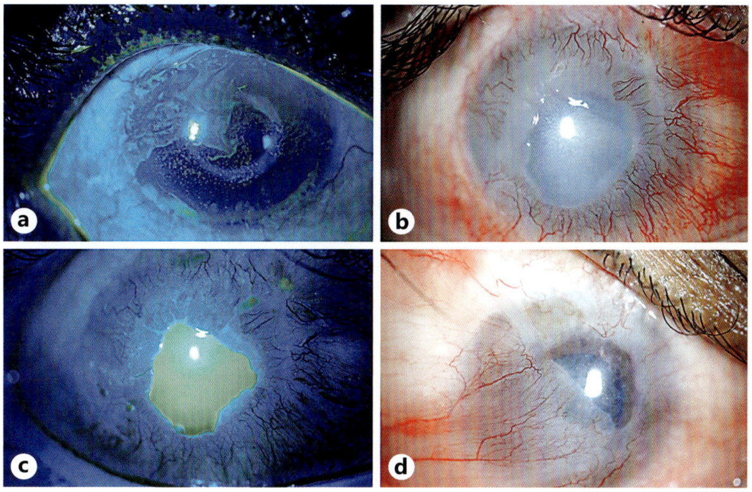

Fig. 22. Examples of limbal stem cell deficiency (LSCD). **a** Conjunctivalization, a hallmark of LSCD, of the cornea in an eye with partial LSCD. **b** Chemical burn with total LSCD, fibrovascular pannus and a central persistent epithelial defect. **c** Fluorescein-stained epithelial defect shown in (**c**). **d** Total LSCD with fibrovascular pannus on the cornea.

unilateral or bilateral and as partial (visual axis affected or spared) or total. The evaluation of the thickness and the clarity of the corneal stroma underlying the fibrovascular pannus, the visual potential by electrophysiological tests, and the intraocular pressure, a workup of the patient for immuno-suppression and HLA typing of the patient and potentially living related donors are required before embarking on treatment.

Treatment Algorithm
Acute Presentation (Chemical Burns)
OS chemical burns are a fairly common cause of LSCD. Immediate assessment may require the instillation of topical anaesthesia. Profuse irrigation, preferably with sterile saline solution, of the conjunctival sac is imperative. Particulate chemical matter should be looked for by double eversion of the upper lid and should be removed. This may require the excision of the conjunctival and subconjunctival tissue in which the material is impregnated. The extent of damage to the conjunctiva, the limbus, the cornea and other anterior and posterior segment structures including the alteration of intraocular pressure should be assessed and documented where possible. The burn should be graded using a standard grading system [56, 57].

Initial conservative management consists of the following: prophylactic antibiotic drops; sodium citrate 10% (4–6 times a day) as a potent inhibitor of neutrophils (proteases); sodium ascorbate drops 5%, although these drops cause severe stinging sensation and may not always be tolerated; frequent application of lubricating drops and topical steroid drops like prednisolone 0.5–1%. Steroids are to be used with caution, as they can aggravate melting. The authors' practice is to use steroids to treat inflammation in the immediate stage of a chemical burn and to watch carefully, reducing the frequency or stopping steroid treatment altogether when any sign of melting of the cornea is seen. Mydriatic/cycloplegic agents are also needed, but sympathomimetic agents should be avoided, as they can aggravate limbal ischaemia. Oral ascorbic acid 2 g/day helps to restore the aqueous ascorbic acid level, which plummets after a chemical burn. Oral tetracycline (doxycycline 100 mg/day) acts as a protease inhibitor and delays or prevents stromal melting. If the eye pressure is high, oral acetazolamide is preferred to topical antiglaucoma agents on account of the multitude of drops that are being used.

When a sector of the limbal epithelium is present, epithelium growing from this sector is

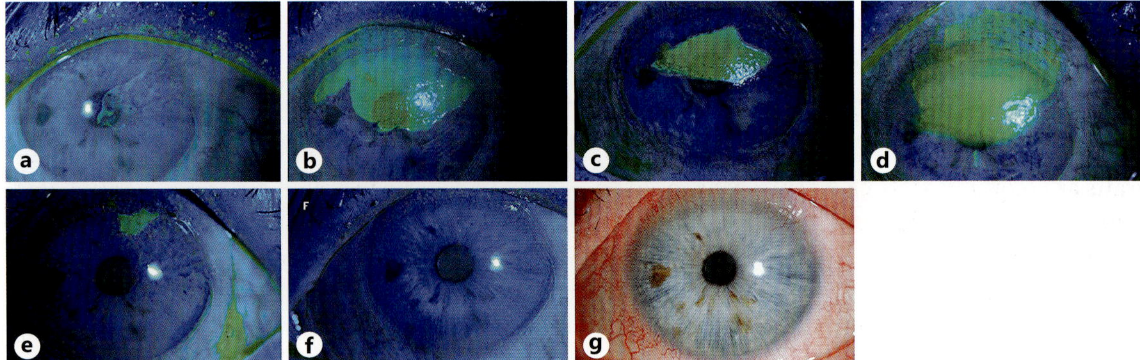

Fig. 23. Sequential sector conjunctival epitheliectomy (SSCE) in partial LSCD with conjunctivalization of the cornea. **a** The conjunctivalized area of the cornea shows late fluorescein staining. **b** The abnormal epithelium on the cornea is 'brushed' away under topical anaesthesia at the slit lamp. **c** After 24 hours, the corneal epithelial defect created by SSCE was healing, but there was encroachment of conjunctival epithelium superiorly. **d** The unwanted epithelium is 'brushed' away via SSCE. **e** After an additional 24 hours, the corneal epithelium is seen to re-establish cover over most of the cornea, particularly over the visual axis. **f, g** Normal corneal epithelial cover has been re-established as seen by fluorescein staining (not late staining (**f**)) and direct illumination (**g**).

Fig. 24. Limbal transplantation.
a Donor site of autolimbal grafts. Two clock hours of limbus and peripheral cornea with 3 mm of adjacent conjunctiva were taken. The conjunctival defect was closed by mobilising the surrounding conjunctiva. **b** An allograft from a living related donor is sutured to the superior and inferior limbus of the recipient eye. **c** An allolimbal (cadaver donor) graft is placed all around the recipient limbus. **d** The same eye as shown in (**c**) after fluorescein staining. The epithelium of the corneal graft and the allolimbal graft were intact.

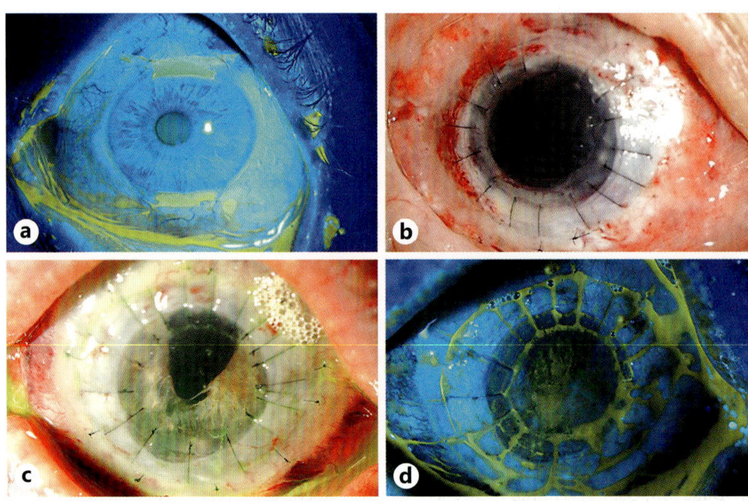

encouraged, while any epithelium coming onto the cornea from the conjunctiva is scraped away daily. This procedure is termed sequential sector conjunctival epitheliectomy (fig. 23a–g). This process allows the cornea to be completely covered by corneal epithelium. When the entire limbus is involved, the conjunctival epithelium should be allowed to cover the cornea, as we believe that any epithelial cover is better than no epithelial cover. In cases in which no epithelialization is observed, one may resort to an AM transplantation, which may reduce the ocular inflammation and may help epithelial migration. Autologous and living related donor limbal SC transplantation is not contemplated until the inflammation has completely subsided and the OS has stabilized, which may take up to 18 months [44]. Grafts performed in the immediate and intermediate stages of chemical burns or during the presence of active inflammation (in other OS disorders) are at high risk of failure. If limbal grafts are required, only cadaver grafts should be considered, as autologous grafts (in unilateral damage) and living related grafts are precious and should be reserved for visual rehabilitation when the inflammation has settled.

In established cases (late-stage chemical burn or inflammatory surface disease) in which there is partial LSCD and the visual axis is not involved, the vision is usually good (potentially requiring a rigid gas permeable lens or mini scleral lens), and only lubricating eye drops may be required. For partial LSCD in which the visual axis is involved, sequential sector conjunctival epitheliectomy is indicated. For total unilateral cases, autolimbal transplantation is the treatment of choice, and for total bilateral cases, allolimbal, cadaver or living related donor transplantation is indicated (fig. 24a–d). AM as a patch or a graft is often a useful adjunct therapy. Ex vivo expanded cell sheets of limbal, oral mucosal or conjunctival epithelium on amnion, fibrin or other substrates are increasingly being used [58–60].

Associated lid abnormalities, symblephara (buccal mucosa grafts), glaucoma and cataracts should ideally be dealt with prior to undertaking OS restorative surgery. When a corneal graft is needed, it is best done as a second procedure after the OS has been restored. When an intumescent cataract is associated with increased pressure, corneal grafting may become a necessity if a dense fibrovascular pannus or corneal scar precludes the visualization of the interior of the eye. In most instances of allolimbal transplantation, long-term immunosuppression is required. The outcomes of autologous grafts are the best, whilst those of cadaver donor grafts are the worst.

References

1   Thoft RA: Role of the ocular surface in destructive corneal disease. Trans Ophthalmol Soc U K 1978;98:339–342.
2   Paulsen F: Functional anatomy and immunological interactions of ocular surface and adnexa. Dev Ophthalmol 2008; 41:21–35.
3   Conrad GW, Funderburgh JL: Eye development and the appearance and maintenance of corneal transparency. Trans Kans Acad Sci 1992;95:34–38.
4   Dana MR, Qian Y, Hamrah P: Twenty-five-year panorama of corneal immunology: emerging concepts in the immunopathogenesis of microbial keratitis, peripheral ulcerative keratitis, and corneal transplant rejection. Cornea 2000; 19:625–643.
5   Knop E, Knop N: Anatomy and immunology of the ocular surface. Chem Immunol Allergy 2007;92:36–49.
6   Dua HS, Miri A, Alomar T, Yeung AM, Said DG: The role of limbal stem cells in corneal epithelial maintenance: testing the dogma. Ophthalmology 2009;116: 856–863.
7   Miri A, Al-Aqaba M, Otri AM, Fares U, Said DG, et al: In vivo confocal microscopic features of normal limbus. Br J Ophthalmol 2012;96:530–536.
8   Miri A, Alomar T, Nubile M, Al-Aqaba M, Lanzini M, et al: In vivo confocal microscopic findings in patients with limbal stem cell deficiency. Br J Ophthalmol 2012;96:523–529.
9   Nubile M, Lanzini M, Miri A, Pocobelli A, Calienno R, et al: In vivo confocal microscopy in diagnosis of limbal stem cell deficiency. Am J Ophthalmol 2013; 155:220–232.
10 Dua HS, Joseph A, Shanmuganathan VA, Jones RE: Stem cell differentiation and the effects of deficiency. Eye (Lond) 2003;17:877–885.
11 Dua HS: The conjunctiva in corneal epithelial wound healing. Br J Ophthalmol 1998;82:1407–1411.
12 Dua HS, Forrester JV: Clinical patterns of corneal epithelial wound healing. Am J Ophthalmol 1987;104:481–489.
13 Dua H, Yeung A, Said DG: Ocular surface stem cells: science and surgery; in Perez VL, Scorsetti DH, Gomes JAP (eds): Stem Cells in Ophthalmology. New Delhi, India, Jaypee Highlights Medical Publishers, 2015, pp 67–79.
14 Al-Aqaba MA, Fares U, Suleman H, Lowe J, Dua HS: Architecture and distribution of human corneal nerves. Br J Ophthalmol 2010;94:784–789.
15 Butler TK, Dua HS, Edwards R, Lowe JS: In vitro model of infectious crystalline keratopathy: tissue architecture determines pattern of microbial spread. Invest Ophthalmol Vis Sci 2001;42:1243–1246.

16 Behrens A, Doyle JJ, Stern L, Chuck RS, McDonnell PJ, et al: Dysfunctional tear syndrome: a Delphi approach to treatment recommendations. Cornea 2006; 25:900–907.

17 Research in dry eye: report of the Research Subcommittee of the International Dry Eye WorkShop (2007). Ocul Surf 2007;5:179–193.

18 Fraunfelder FT, Sciubba JJ, Mathers WD: The role of medications in causing dry eye. J Ophthalmol 2012;2012: 285851.

19 Finis D, Konig C, Hayajneh J, Borrelli M, Schrader S, et al: Six-month effects of a thermodynamic treatment for MGD and implications of meibomian gland atrophy. Cornea 2014;33:1265–1270.

20 Foulks GN, Borchman D, Yappert M, Kakar S: Topical azithromycin and oral doxycycline therapy of meibomian gland dysfunction: a comparative clinical and spectroscopic pilot study. Cornea 2013;32:44–53.

21 Schrage N, Frentz M, Spoeler F: The Ex Vivo Eye Irritation Test (EVEIT) in evaluation of artificial tears: purite-preserved versus unpreserved eye drops. Graefes Arch Clin Exp Ophthalmol 2012;250:1333–1340.

22 Baxter SA, Laibson PR: Punctal plugs in the management of dry eyes. Ocul Surf 2004;2:255–265.

23 Schultz C: Safety and efficacy of cyclosporine in the treatment of chronic dry eye. Ophthalmol Eye Dis 2014;6:37–42.

24 Nanavaty MA, Long M, Malhotra R: Transdermal androgen patches in evaporative dry eye syndrome with androgen deficiency: a pilot study. Br J Ophthalmol 2014;98:567–569.

25 Alomar T, Matthew M, Donald F, Maharajan S, Dua HS: In vivo confocal microscopy in the diagnosis and management of acanthamoeba keratitis showing new cystic forms. Clin Exp Ophthalmol 2009;37:737–739.

26 Dart JK, Saw VP, Kilvington S: Acanthamoeba keratitis: diagnosis and treatment update 2009. Am J Ophthalmol 2009;148:487–499.e2.

27 Dua HS, Otri AM, Said DG, Faraj LA: The 'up-down' sign of acute ocular surface drug toxicity. Br J Ophthalmol 2012;96:1439–1440.

28 Dua HS, Aralikatti A, Said DG: Rapid diagnosis of Acanthamoeba keratitis. Br J Ophthalmol 2009;93:1555–1556.

29 Claerhout I, Goegebuer A, Van Den Broecke C, Kestelyn P: Delay in diagnosis and outcome of Acanthamoeba keratitis. Graefes Arch Clin Exp Ophthalmol 2004;242:648–653.

30 Schuster FL, Visvesvara GS: Opportunistic amoebae: challenges in prophylaxis and treatment. Drug Resist Updat 2004; 7:41–51.

31 Kimberlin DW, Whitley RJ: Antiviral therapy of HSV-1 and -2; in Arvin A, Campadelli-Fiume G, Mocarski E, Moore PS, Roizman B, et al (eds): Human Herpesviruses: Biology, Therapy, and Immunoprophylaxis. Cambridge, Cambridge University Press, 2007.

32 Sacchetti M, Lambiase A: Diagnosis and management of neurotrophic keratitis. Clin Ophthalmol 2014;8:571–579.

33 Rowe AM, St Leger AJ, Jeon S, Dhaliwal DK, Knickelbein JE, et al: Herpes keratitis. Prog Retin Eye Res 2013;32:88–101.

34 Thomas PA, Teresa PA, Theodore J, Geraldine P: PCR for the molecular diagnosis of mycotic keratitis. Expert Rev Mol Diagn 2012;12:703–718.

35 Said DG, Otri M, Miri A, Kailasanathan A, Khatib T, et al: The challenge of fungal keratitis. Br J Ophthalmol 2011;95: 1623–1624.

36 Sharma N, Agarwal P, Sinha R, Titiyal JS, Velpandian T, et al: Evaluation of intrastromal voriconazole injection in recalcitrant deep fungal keratitis: case series. Br J Ophthalmol 2011;95:1735–1737.

37 Xie L, Zhai H, Shi W: Penetrating keratoplasty for corneal perforations in fungal keratitis. Cornea 2007;26:158–162.

38 Gicquel JJ, Bejjani RA, Ellies P, Mercie M, Dighiero P: Amniotic membrane transplantation in severe bacterial keratitis. Cornea 2007;26:27–33.

39 Mencucci R, Menchini U, Dei R: Antimicrobial activity of antibiotic-treated amniotic membrane: an in vitro study. Cornea 2006;25:428–431.

40 Said DG, Elalfy MS, Gatzioufas Z, El-Zakzouk ES, Hassan MA, et al: Collagen cross-linking with photoactivated riboflavin (PACK-CXL) for the treatment of advanced infectious keratitis with corneal melting. Ophthalmology 2014;121: 1377–1382.

41 Galicia-Carreon J, Santacruz C, Hong E, Jimenez-Martinez MC: The ocular surface: from physiology to the ocular allergic diseases. Rev Alerg Mex 2013;60: 172–183.

42 Chang JH, McCluskey PJ: Ocular cicatricial pemphigoid: manifestations and management. Curr Allergy Asthma Rep 2005;5:333–338.

43 Saw VP, Dart JK: Ocular mucous membrane pemphigoid: diagnosis and management strategies. Ocul Surf 2008;6: 128–142.

44 Dua HS, Miri A, Said DG: Contemporary limbal stem cell transplantation – a review. Clin Exp Ophthalmol 2010;38: 104–117.

45 Power WJ, Ghoraishi M, Merayo-Lloves J, Neves RA, Foster CS: Analysis of the acute ophthalmic manifestations of the erythema multiforme/Stevens-Johnson syndrome/toxic epidermal necrolysis disease spectrum. Ophthalmology 1995; 102:1669–1676.

46 Sethuraman G, Sharma VK, Pahwa P, Khetan P: Causative drugs and clinical outcome in Stevens Johnson syndrome (SJS), toxic epidermal necrolysis (TEN), and SJS-TEN overlap in children. Indian J Dermatol 2012;57:199–200.

47 Pichler WJ, Naisbitt DJ, Park BK: Immune pathomechanism of drug hypersensitivity reactions. J Allergy Clin Immunol 2011;127:S74–S81.

48 De Rojas MV, Dart JK, Saw VP: The natural history of Stevens Johnson syndrome: patterns of chronic ocular disease and the role of systemic immunosuppressive therapy. Br J Ophthalmol 2007;91:1048–1053.

49 Kolomeyer AM, Do BK, Tu Y, Chu DS: Placement of ProKera in the management of ocular manifestations of acute Stevens-Johnson syndrome in an outpatient. Eye Contact Lens 2013;39:e7–e11.

50 Kawasaki S, Nishida K, Sotozono C, Quantock AJ, Kinoshita S: Conjunctival inflammation in the chronic phase of Stevens-Johnson syndrome. Br J Ophthalmol 2000;84:1191–1193.

51 Bernauer W, Broadway DC, Wright P: Chronic progressive conjunctival cicatrisation. Eye (Lond) 1993;7:371–378.

52 Bernauer W, Elder MJ, Leonard JN, Wright P, Dart JK: The value of biopsies in the evaluation of chronic progressive conjunctival cicatrisation. Graefes Arch Clin Exp Ophthalmol 1994;232:533–537.

53 Khalili B, Bahna SL: Pathogenesis and recent therapeutic trends in Stevens-Johnson syndrome and toxic epidermal necrolysis. Ann Allergy Asthma Immunol 2006;97:272–280; quiz 281–283, 320.

54 Foster CS, Fong LP, Azar D, Kenyon KR: Episodic conjunctival inflammation after Stevens-Johnson syndrome. Ophthalmology 1988;95:453–462.

55 Dua HS, Forrester JV: The corneoscleral limbus in human corneal epithelial wound healing. Am J Ophthalmol 1990; 110:646–656.

56 Dua HS, King AJ, Joseph A: A new classification of ocular surface burns. Br J Ophthalmol 2001;85:1379–1383.

57 Roper-Hall MJ: Thermal and chemical burns. Trans Ophthalmol Soc UK 1965; 85:631–653.

58 Pathak M, Cholidis S, Haug K, Shahdadfar A, Moe MC, et al: Clinical transplantation of ex vivo expanded autologous limbal epithelial cells using a culture medium with human serum as single supplement: a retrospective case series. Acta Ophthalmol 2013;91:769–775.

59 Higa K, Shimazaki J: Recent advances in cultivated epithelial transplantation. Cornea 2008;27(suppl 1):S41–S47.

60 Kolli S, Ahmad S, Mudhar HS, Meeny A, Lako M, et al: Successful application of ex vivo expanded human autologous oral mucosal epithelium for the treatment of total bilateral limbal stem cell deficiency. Stem Cells 2014;32:2135–2146.

Harminder S. Dua
Academic Ophthalmology Section, Division of Clinical Neuroscience
University of Nottingham
NG7 2UH Nottingham (UK)
E-Mail profdua@gmail.com

Güell JL (ed): Cornea. ESASO Course Series. Basel, Karger, 2015, vol 6, pp 26–38
DOI: 10.1159/000381490

Surgical Management of Post-Keratoplasty Astigmatism

Rudy M.M.A. Nuijts · Soraya M.R. Jonker · Isabelle E.Y. Saelens

University Eye Clinic Maastricht, Maastricht University Medical Center, Maastricht, The Netherlands

Abstract

Penetrating keratoplasty (PK) with a clear graft results in improved visual acuity. However, visual acuity can be limited by significant postoperative astigmatism. There are currently several treatment options for post-PK astigmatism. Because of its moderate effectiveness and unpredictable outcomes, incisional surgery can be used to prime the cornea before laser correction is applied. Laser ablation with photorefractive keratectomy or laser-assisted subepithelial keratectomy has been proven to be equally effective in terms of the correction of refraction. The refractive results with laser in situ keratomileusis seem similar to those with surface ablation, but flap complications can occur. While implantation of either phakic or pseudophakic toric intraocular lenses (IOLs) can generate excellent refractive results, some preoperative thought is required. Phakic toric IOLs cause more endothelial cell loss in post-PK patients than in people with virgin eyes, and this cell loss can eventually result in re-PK if corneal decompensation occurs. Fortunately, phakic toric IOLs can be removed without much difficulty. In patients scheduled for pseudophakic toric IOL implantation, it is very important to consider if re-PK is likely to occur in the future. If so, introducing a phakic IOL on top of the implanted monofocal pseudophakic IOL might be a more preferable option.

Introduction

Penetrating keratoplasty (PK) with a clear graft results in improved visual acuity. However, visual acuity can be limited by significant postoperative astigmatism. Research shows that regular and irregular astigmatism occur in 24% and 72% of PK patients, respectively [1]. Thirty percent of patients suffer from astigmatism of more than 5 D. Therefore, post-PK astigmatism is a common problem. As Brooks et al. [2] proved in 1996, we now know that anisometropia or astigmatism of more than 3–4 D is generally not tolerated by patients. Negative effects on high-grade binocular interaction seem to be related to the degree of anisometropia [2].

Several known causes of astigmatism after PK are described in the literature. Causes such as dif-

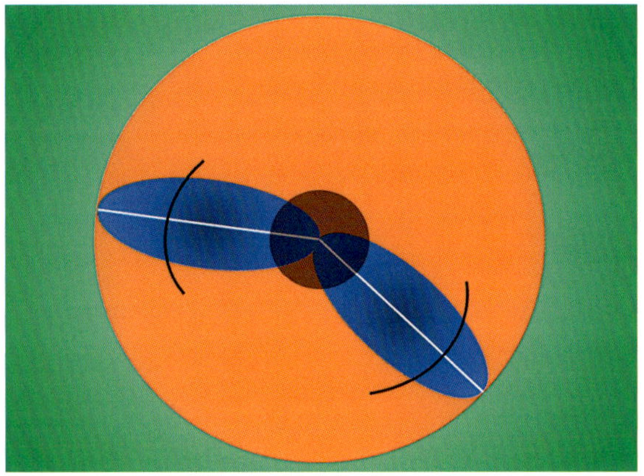

Fig. 1. Arcuate keratotomy, schematic.

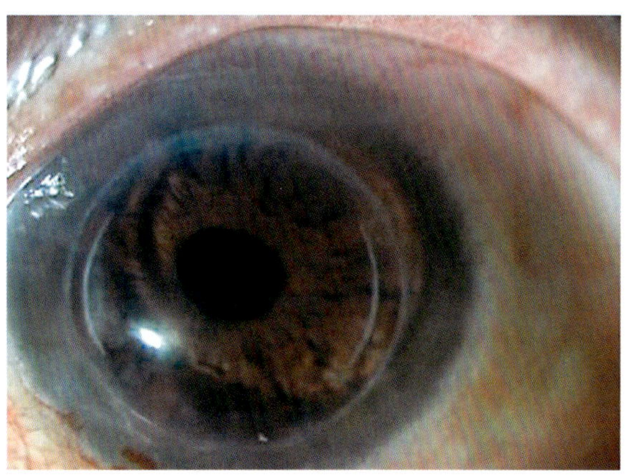

Fig. 2. Arcuate keratotomy after penetrating keratoplasty.

ferences between the donor and the host in size, thickness and shape, eccentric placement, irregular scarring at the host junction and asymmetric tractional forces (i.e. sutures) are reported by van Rij et al. and Kerenyi et al. [3, 4].

Initial treatment of residual refractive disorders consists of spectacle correction or contact lens fitting. Several types of contact lens designs are currently available to correct high levels of both regular and irregular astigmatism [5, 6]. From 20 to 40% of all PK patients and from 40 to 50% of PK-for-keratoconus patients need to be fitted with contact lenses [5, 7].

This chapter will discuss the different interventions available to patients who are contact lens intolerant or who have excessive regular or irregular astigmatism.

Relaxing Incisions and Compression Sutures

Application of relaxing incisions (RIs) (i.e. arcuate keratotomy) or compression sutures (CSs) can adjust astigmatism of as much as 4–5 D in patients with congenital astigmatism. RIs are performed in the steep corneal meridian (fig. 1), whereas CSs are placed in the flat corneal meridian [8, 9]. A combined procedure can also be per-

formed in order to optimize astigmatic correction in those with high levels of astigmatism [8, 9].

Unfortunately, predictability in transplanted corneas is very poor, with minimal effect on spherical equivalent (fig. 2). The use of this technique is difficult because normograms used on patients with congenital astigmatism do not apply to post-PK patients. Multiple studies show that the astigmatic effect of the incision is proportional to the preoperative cylinder [8–11]. RIs can be performed at different sites (host, interface, or graft) at varying incision depth and length. Traditional RIs are performed manually with a diamond knife, resulting in variable incision depth and length as well as a risk of corneal perforation during surgery.

The results of several studies of RIs and CSs are summarized in table 1 [8, 10–16].

A total of 217 patients participated in studies about RIs with or without CSs after PK. Three different incision locations were described: the graft [11, 12, 14, 15], the interface between the host cornea and the graft [8, 16] and the host cornea [10, 13]. An overall reduction in refractive cylinder, varying from 45 to 72%, was seen. Complications occurred in 4 studies and consisted of graft rejection (1/34 [8] and 2/40 [15] patients) and perforation (1/39, [11] 1/40 [15] and 1/26 [16] patients).

Authors	N	Treatment	Location	Refractive cylinder, mean ± SD			Complication
				pre-op, D	post-op, D	reduction, %	
Hjortdal and Ehlers, 1998 [12]	21	RI	Graft	7.0	3.3	54	None
Koay et al., 2000 [8]	34	RI and CS	Interface	9.1±4.4	3.6±1.9	61	1/34 graft rejection
Wilkins et al., 2005 [10]	20	RI	Host	−11.0	−3.0	72	None
Bochmann and Schipper, 2006 [13]	11	RI	Host	9.2	3.4	46	None
Geggel, 2006 [14]	26	RI	Graft	8.7±2.4	3.3±1.7	63	None
Poole and Ficker, 2006 [11]	39	RI	Graft	9.1	4.9	47	1/39 perforation
Hoffart et al., 2007 [15]	40	RI	Graft	8.8±3.6	4.9±2.5	45	1/40 perforation 2/40 rejection
Fares et al., 2013 [16]	26	RI and CS	Interface	9.6±2.9	4.4±2.5	58	1 microperforation

D = Diopters; RI = relaxing incisions; CS = compressive sutures.

New treatment options with the femtosecond (FS) laser allow the surgeon to accurately determine the incision depth during surgery. However, when placing the laser markings on the applanated corneal surface, there is no clear view of the host-graft interface, resulting in imperfect alignment of the cut and the host-graft interface.

Five studies reported the results of FS-RIs in post-PK patients (table 2) [17–20]. The results for a total of 82 patients showed an overall reduction in refractive cylinder varying from 36 to 66%, with perforation occurring in 17% of patients in just one study [19]. Graft rejection was not reported in any of the studies mentioned in table 2. FS-RIs seemed to induce less perforations, but the refractive cylinder results seemed similar to the results using manual RIs (table 1, 2).

Even though studies show improvement in refractive cylinder results and astigmatic correc-tion, it seems that optimal results can be obtained when RIs and CSs are used to prime the post-PK patient for additional laser refractive surgery. Laser refractive surgery on the post-PK patient will be discussed further down this chapter.

Wedge Excision

Traditional manual wedge excision can be applied to patients with high levels of astigmatism. Like manual RIs, the manual wedge excision is extremely prone to intraoperative perforation. In addition to this major risk, it is difficult to remove the appropriate amount of tissue required for optimal astigmatic correction. In order to improve the safety as well as the reproducibility of refractive results, Ghanem et al. [21] reported on the use of the FS laser to perform wedge excisions (fig. 3). Their case report described a simple

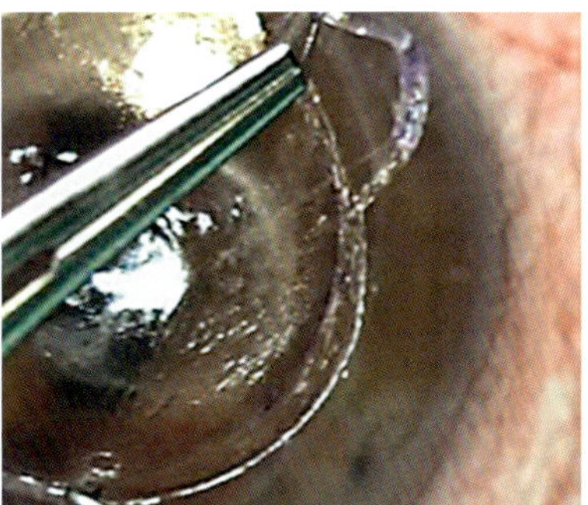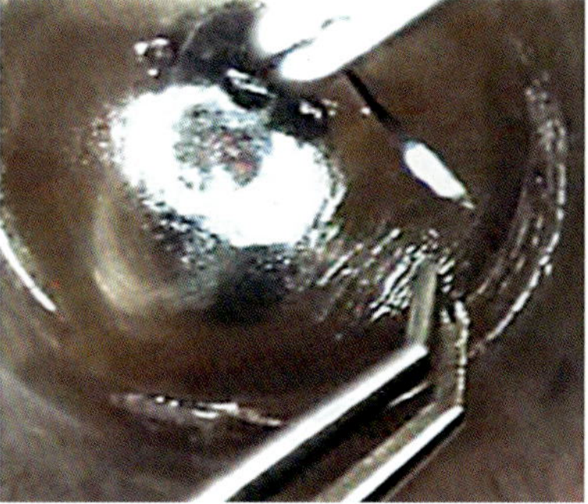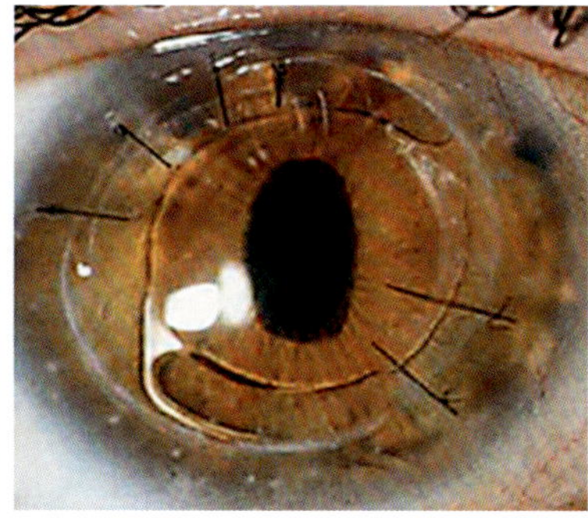

Fig. 3. Wedge excision with a femtosecond laser [21].

Table 2. Results for FS laser-assisted relaxing incisions in patients after PK

Authors	N	Method	Refractive cylinder, mean ± SD			BCVA loss of ≥2 Snellen lines, %	Complication	
			pre-op, D	post-op, D	reduction, %		perforation, %	over-correction, %
Cleary et al., 2013 [17]	6	FS Beveled	9.8±2.9	4.5±3.2	57	0	0	NR
Kumar et al., 2010 [18]	34	FS	7.5±2.7	4.8±3.3	36	0	0	24
Nubile et al., 2009 [19]	12	FS	7.2±3.1	2.4±1.6	66	0	17	NR
Hoffart et al., 2009 [20]	10	FS	8.6±3.0	3.9±2.4	55	20	0	NR
	10	Hanna	6.7±2.1	4.7±2.4	30	0	10	NR
Bahar, 2008 [66]	20	FS	7.8±2.4	3.6±2.2	54	0	0	25
	20	Manual	7.8±3.1	4.6±3.0	41	0	15	30

D = Diopters; BCVA = best-corrected visual acuity; FS = femtosecond; NR = not reported.

formula that allows the FS laser to make an easier, more controlled, and more precise excision of tissue in terms of width, length, and depth, probably leading to improved reproducibility of the technique in patients with astigmatism from 6.3 to 20 D [21].

Femtosecond Laser-Assisted Intrastromal Corneal Ring Segment Implantation

Lisa et al. [22] published the results on their 2013 study of 32 post-PK eyes that underwent FS laser-assisted Ferrara ring segment implantation (fig. 4). Their results looked promising, with significantly improved uncorrected distance visual acuity (UDVA) (p < 0.0001) and corrected distance visual acuity (CDVA) (p < 0.0001), including a UDVA of ≥20/40 in 40.6% of eyes and a CDVA of ≥20/25 in 56.2% of eyes [22]. Loss of more than 2 lines of CDVA did not occur in any patient; the 6-month safety index was 1.20; and both spherical equivalent and astigmatism were significantly reduced after implantation of the Ferrara ring segments [22].

No further studies have been published with regard to the use of Ferrara ring segments for the treatment of post-PK astigmatism.

Authors	N	Refractive cylinder, mean ± SD			BCVA loss of ≥2 Snellen lines, %	UCVA ≥20/40, %	Complication
		pre-op, D	post-op, D	reduction, %			
Campos, 1992 [23]	12	7.0±3.6	4.3±2.9	39	0	17	Regression
Lazzaro, 1996 [24]	7	5.3±2.0	2.8±1.6	48	29	0	2/7 loss BCVA
Amm et al., 1996 [25]	16	5.7	2.9	38–57	14	14	4/16 haze II
Tuunanen et al., 1997 [26]	10	6.0±2.3	4.3±2.4	48	40	10	4/10 haze II
Bansal, 1999 [27]	10	5.8	3.2	45	0	0	5/10 haze II
Bilgihan et al., 2000 [28]	16	5.6±2.9	3.2±1.7	43	6.3	25	6/16 haze II-III 2/16 loss BCVA

D = Diopters; UCVA = uncorrected visual acuity; BCVA = best-corrected visual acuity.

Excimer Laser Ablations

Laser ablative techniques like photorefractive keratectomy (PRK), laser-assisted subepithelial keratectomy (LASEK) and laser in situ keratomileusis (LASIK) are on the rise as methods to correct astigmatism after PK. The primary goal of these treatments is the correction of refractive errors in a way that enables correction with spectacles or contact lenses.

Photorefractive Keratectomy/ Photoastigmatic Refractive Keratectomy

PRK, sometimes noted as photoastigmatic refractive keratectomy (PARK), has been investigated for the correction of post-PK astigmatism in several older series with small patient groups (n = 7–16) [23–28]. Similar to the previously mentioned treatment methods, the treatment effect of PRK on the transplanted eye differs from that on the virgin eye. This is the result of differences in wound healing in the corneal graft. Table 3 presents the refractive and visual results from the series on PRK in post-PK astigmatism in a total of 71 patients. Reduction of the refractive cylinder varied

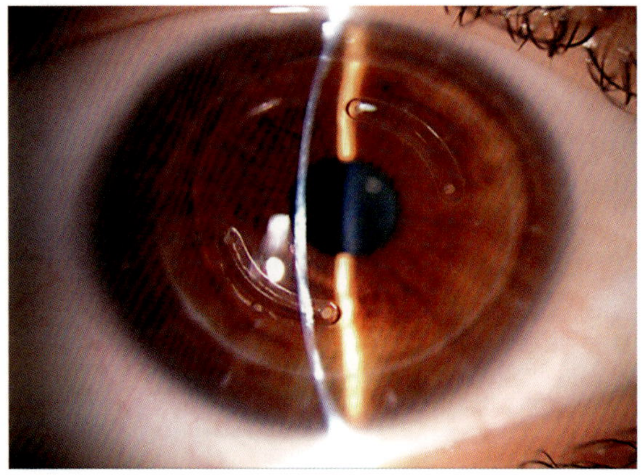

Fig. 4. Ferrara intrastromal ring segments [22].

from 38 to 57%, postoperative uncorrected visual acuity was ≥20/40 in 0–25% of patients and loss of ≥2 Snellen lines of best-corrected visual acuity (BCVA) occurred in 0–40% of patients [23–28].

Up to 50% of patients with PRK after PK experience corneal haze formation (fig. 5) [27], which could possibly cause irregular astigmatism and a higher rate of refractive regression (table 3).

New developments in PRK application consist of topography-guided excimer laser ablation and the modulation of wound healing by

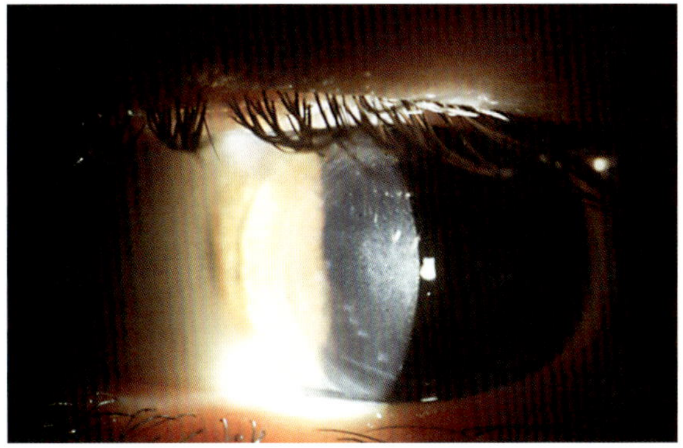

Fig. 5. Grade III haze after photorefractive keratectomy.

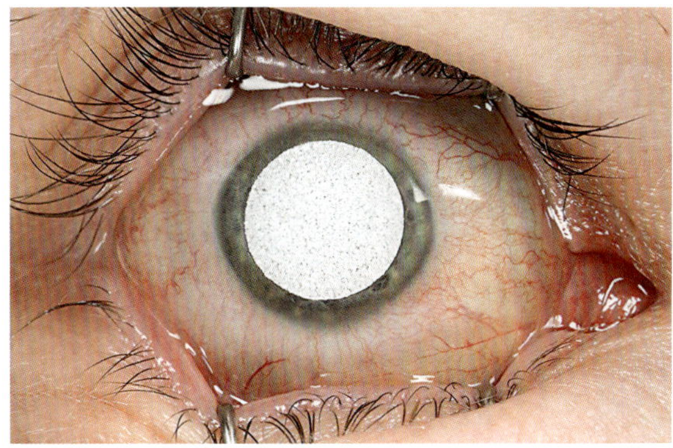

Fig. 6. Mitomycin C application after laser ablation.

applying mitomycin C (MMC) during surgery [29, 30]. Hjortdal et al. [29] described a study of 16 eyes that underwent topography-guided PRK without MMC application. BCVA improved significantly (p < 0.05), but no significant change in coma, spherical aberrations or higher-order aberrations (HOAs) was seen. Grade III corneal haze requiring additional surgery occurred in 4/16 (25%) eyes [29]. No results on PRK with MMC post-PK are currently published, but a study of PRK with MMC post-deep anterior lamellar keratoplasty showed no corneal haze or regression (0/10) in the 10-month follow-up period [30].

ment for a maximum of –7 D of astigmatism. Two subgroups could be distinguished: with and without MMC application (n = 4 and n = 12, respectively). Spherical equivalent was within 1 D of intended correction in 62.5% of patients; mean astigmatism was reduced by 57%, and HOAs significantly decreased, as well [32].

Post-PK patients are prone to haze formation and refractive regression. The results of this study show good refractive stability in both subgroups. Haze did occur but seemed to be less in the eyes that received intra-operative MMC [32].

Currently, no consensus has been reached on the optimal dose and exposure time for MMC (fig. 6).

Laser-Assisted Subepithelial Keratectomy

One retrospective comparative study of LASEK versus PRK included a total of 85 laser-ablated eyes. Fifty-three eyes underwent LASEK, and thirty-two underwent PRK; MMC was not administered in this study [31]. No significant difference between the treatments was seen with respect to any of the outcome measures [31].

Rajan et al. [32] reported the results of a study on topography-guided LASEK with application of MMC in patients with irregular astigmatism after PK. Preoperative lower-order aberrations and HOAs were linked to customized laser treat-

Laser in situ Keratomileusis

It is suggested in the literature that LASIK is gaining ground on PRK as a treatment for post-PK astigmatism. LASIK has several advantages over PRK, such as swift visual rehabilitation, reduced corneal scarring, minimal regression risk and the ability to treat a wider range of refractive errors [33].

In order to optimize wound healing after PK, the predominant rhetoric advises corneal/refractive surgeons to withhold LASIK from post-PK patients for at least 1 year and to wait at least 3 months after suture removal.

Table 4. Results of LASIK in patients after PKP

Authors	N	Procedure	Redo, %	Refractive cylinder, mean ± SD			UCVA ≥20/40, %	BCVA, %	
				pre-op, D	post-op, D	reduction, %		loss of ≥2 Snellen lines	gain of ≥2 Snellen lines
Donnenfeld et al., 1999 [34]	22	LASIK	9.1	3.6±1.7	1.3±1.0	55	36	4.3	26
Webber et al., 1999 [41]	26	LASIK	NR	6.6	3.4	48.7	28	0	12
	26/14	LASIK/AK	NR	10.3	2.4	76.3			
Rashad, 2000 [35]	19	LASIK	53	9.2±1.9	1.1±0.3	88	74	0	42
Kwitko et al., 2001 [36]	14	LASIK	43	5.4±2.1	2.8±2.4	47.5	29	7.1	21
Malecha and Holland, 2002 [37]	20	LASIK	NR	4.1±1.7	1.2±1.1	69.9	30	5	0
Barraquer and Rodriguez-Barraquer, 2004 [38]	46	LASIK	15	3.7	1.7	53.8	33	6.5	36.9
Buzard et al., 2004 [39]	26	LASIK	39	2.7±2.3	1.1±0.7	60.9	86	0	5
Hardten et al., 2004 [40]	57/15	LASIK/AK	9	4.7±2.2	1.9±1.4	58.5	43	16	28

D = Diopters; UCVA = uncorrected visual acuity; BCVA = best-corrected visual acuity; AK = arcuate keratotomy; NR = not reported.

The efficacy of LASIK is limited by its dependence on corneal graft thickness and the amount of refractive error suitable for correction. Furthermore, wound apposition of the graft and the host cornea is of the utmost importance to prevent override or underride of the flap. Adequate endothelial cell counts are required, as well, in order to prevent the development of fluid pockets in the interface [33].

Even when all of the abovementioned factors are taken into consideration, complications still occur. Wound dehiscence, for one, can be induced by the high vacuum pressure during LASIK. Flap complications such as button holes can occur in steep corneas, and a high rate of enhancements (up to 53%) has been reported in previous studies [33–40]. Patients who received PK because of keratoconus are at risk for developing recurrent keratoconus in the graft; a flap created in an ectatic recipient bed may reactivate the progressive corneal ectasia witnessed in keratoconus. The creation of the flap itself can induce diminished corneal sensation, resulting in surface problems like sicca or a neurotrophic ulcus.

Various studies on LASIK for post-PK astigmatism are presented in table 4. We found a reduction in refractive cylinder varying from 47.5 to 88% in a total of 8 conducted studies [34–41]. Uncorrected visual acuity of ≥20/40, loss of ≥2 Snellen lines of BCVA and gain of ≥2 Snellen lines of BCVA was achieved in 29–86%, 0–16% and 0–36.9% of patients, respectively [34–41].

Because it was suspected that solely executing lamellar keratotomy could have a refractive effect, a modified LASIK procedure was executed in three studies [42–44].

This so-called two-step or two-stage procedure consists of (1) creating the corneal flap and (2) performing the excimer laser ablation several months later [43]. Studies suggested that the two-step approach results in better predictability as well as a better and more precise refractive outcome. When looking at the results of these studies, the study performed by Kollias et al. [44] showed no significant changes in either the sphere

Table 5. Results for two-step LASIK in patients after PK

Authors	N	1-stage vs. 2-stage	Refractive cylinder, mean ± SD			Spherical equivalent, mean ± SD		
			pre-op, D	post-flap, D	post-ablation, D	pre-op, D	post-flap, D	post-ablation, D
Busin et al., 2001 [42]	9	Lamellar flap	5.0±1.4	3.4±1.3	–	5.4±1.7	4.4±1.7	–
Alio et al., 2004 [43]	11	1-stage	–4.8±1.7	–	–2.4±2.0	–3.5±2.2	–	–0.6±1.6
	11	2-stage	–6.8±2.5	–2.8±1.9	–2.4±1.5	–3.2±3.6	–2.2±2.3	–1.1±1.0
Kollias et al., 2009 [44]	9	2-stage	–7.3±3.6	–6.7±3.7	–2.1±1.8	–4.0±4.8	–4.1±4.6	–1.1±2.4

D = Diopters.

or the cylinder after sole keratotomy. Only the study by Alio et al. [43] implied a refractive effect of keratotomy alone. An overview of the results of these studies is presented in table 5.

It remains unclear if a two-step procedure results in a higher complication rate for epithelial ingrowth, problems with wound healing or flap dislocation.

Toric Phakic Intraocular Lens Implantation: Iris-Fixated

The implantation of toric phakic intraocular lenses (IOLs; pIOLs) offers a major advantage with regard to the treatment of the PK graft. In contrast to the previously mentioned treatment methods, there is no manipulation or laser ablation of the graft, and the iris-fixated (Artisan) lens can be removed if necessary [45].

The Artisan toric IOL is an iris-fixated phakic lens with a power ranging from –3.0 to –20.5 D and +2.0 to +12.0 D (fig. 7). Cylindrical power ranges from 2.0 to 7.5 D and is either in line with or at a 90-degree angle to the haptics.

Moshirfar et al. [46, 47] published two studies on a total of four patients implanted with a toric pIOL for the correction of post-PK astigmatism. Their case reports showed good initial results, but long-term effects and safety and the significance of the refractive results were not studied.

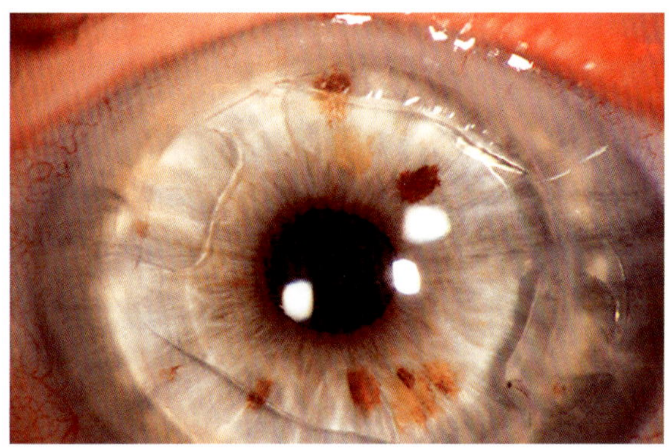

Fig. 7. Toric Artisan after PK.

In 2004, Nuijts et al. [45] reported on the safety and efficacy of Artisan IOL implantation (n = 16). They showed a 78.0 ± 11.5% reduction in the refractive cylinder, which is superior to the results of LASIK post-PK. The follow-up, which was a mean of 8.4 months after Artisan implantation, showed a stable refractive error, no losses in Snellen lines of BCVA and an increase of ≥2 Snellen lines of BCVA in 50% of cases. Reported endothelial cell loss of 7.6 ± 18.9, 21.7 ± 22.3 and 16.6 ± 20.4% was measured at the 3-month, 6-month and final follow-up, respectively. Reversible graft rejection occurred in 1/16 (6.25%) patients [45].

Tahzib et al. studied the long term-effects of Artisan implantation in the eye after PK [48].

This study included a total of 36 eyes and performed follow-up visits lasting up to 4 years (n = 6) with a mean follow-up of 28.5 months (n = 36). Postoperative cylinder was significantly reduced at all time-points (p < 0.001), spherical equivalent decreased from –3.19 ± 4.31 D preoperatively to –1.03 ± 1.20 D at the final follow-up and refractive astigmatism was reduced by 88.8%. Long-term endothelial cell loss was 13.8 ± 18.7% (n = 34), 21.2 ± 21.8% (n = 33), 29.6 ± 27.3% (n = 26), 30.4 ± 32.0% (n = 18) and 34.8 ± 26.3% (n = 6) at, respectively 6 months, 1, 2, 3 and 4 years postoperatively. Irreversible graft rejection occurred in 2/36 patients (5.56%), while 1/36 patients experienced gradual endothelial decompensation (2.78%) [48].

When comparing Artisan implantation between virgin and post-PK eyes, implantation seems to have a more traumatic effect on the corneal endothelium of transplanted patients. While normal adult eyes have an average annual endothelial loss of 0.6% [49], previous studies on endothelial cell loss after PK showed a 34.0 ± 22.0% decrease in year 1, a 7.8% annual decrease in years 3–5 and a 4.2% annual decrease in years 5–10 [50, 51]. It is suggested that the mean endothelial cell loss 5 years post-PK is 59% [50]. This supports the previous assumption that Artisan implantation can have a more traumatic effect on the vulnerable endothelial cells of the graft, resulting in higher endothelial cell loss.

Before implanting an iris-fixated pIOL, the surgeon can rely on preoperative models simulating the position of the pIOL in the eye. These models determine the approximate distance to the corneal endothelium and the crystalline lens, thus preventing pIOL contact as well as minimizing endothelial cell loss [52, 53].

A potential drawback of Artisan toric pIOL implantation is the rather large incision needed for the implantation of the rigid lens. A 5.3 mm incision is necessary to facilitate implantation, which could lead to the interference of surgically induced astigmatism (SIA) with the final refractive results. In a post-PK patient, the corneoscleral tissue may exhibit an unpredictable reaction to manipulation, resulting in a wide variability in SIA, as witnessed in the study by Tahzib et al. [48]. The results of this study suggest not incorporating SIA into the power calculation of the toric pIOL. The more recent Artiflex toric pIOL is foldable, possibly resulting in lower levels of SIA. Unfortunately, no studies of its use in post-PK patients have been published as of yet.

It can be hypothesized that the current inclusion and exclusion criteria for toric pIOLs (i.e. endothelial cell density $\geq$1,000 cells/mm^2, minimal lens-IOL-cornea distance) [54–57] do not have to be applied as strictly as they should for refractive patients. It is important to remember that post-PK patients undergo an operation in order to achieve a refractive error that is correctable by spectacle or contact lens wear. Because Artisan implantation is a reversible procedure, the pIOL can easily be removed if a re-transplant is necessary. A preoperative endothelial cell density of 500 cells/mm^2 should therefore not rule out implantation into the post-PK patient [45].

Toric Phakic Intraocular Lens Implantation: Posterior Chamber

Posterior chamber lenses have not been applied in many studies of the treatment of post-PK astigmatism. One study reported the results of 16 patients implanted with the Visian toric implantable collamer lens (ICL) [58]. The Visian Toric ICL ranges from +10.0 to –18.0 D with a cylindrical power ranging from +1.0 to +6.0 D and is placed in the posterior chamber (fig. 8).

Postoperative refraction was within 1 D of desired refraction in 88% of patients and within 0.5 D in 66.6% of patients. Moreover, 46.6% of patients had a UDVA $\geq$20/40; 80% had a CDVA $\geq$20/40; no patient lost $\geq$2 Snellen lines of BCVA;

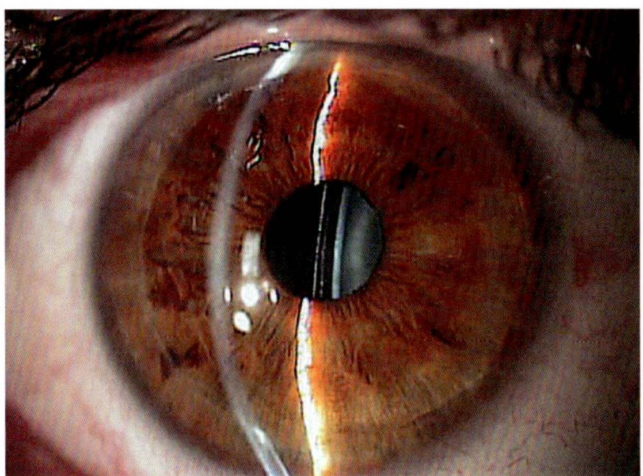

Fig. 8. Visian toric ICL after PK.

and 33.3% of patients gained ≥2 Snellen lines of BCVA [58].

The risks of ICL implantation consist of pupillary block, increased intraocular pressure or cataract induction due to an insufficient distance between the ICL and the crystalline lens [59].

Combined Cataract Surgery

In patients with both cataract and a history of PK, there are several treatment options. First, a standard cataract surgery with implantation of a monofocal pseudophakic IOL can be performed. Second, a toric pseudophakic IOL can be chosen. Finally, a standard cataract surgery with implantation of a monofocal pseudophakic lens can be combined with a separate, reversible toric correction by means of a toric Artisan or Visian toric ICL.

The essential consideration here is whether it is likely that the patient might need a re-PK in the future. A separate toric addition can be removed in such a case. This is especially important because the induced astigmatism will almost certainly differ from the axis and the value of the toric addition already in the eye.

Several different toric IOLs are currently available for implantation (table 6). A series of small studies describe case reports varying from 1 to 7 patients implanted with one of these IOLs as a treatment for their post-PK astigmatism. These results suggest very good refractive outcomes in patients with high astigmatism [60–63].

Viestenz et al. and Wade et al. presented studies of 11 and 21 eyes implanted with toric IOLs after PK, respectively [64, 65]. The 2006 study by Viestenz et al. [64] showed good improvement of refractive astigmatism from 7.0 ± 2.6 D preoperatively to 1.6 ± 1.5 D postoperatively (mean follow-up of 3.5 months), with deviation from the target axis of 4.1 ± 2.9 degrees (0–8 degrees). Graft failure did not occur in any patient, and endothelial loss was limited from 1,300 cells/mm^2 to 1,288 cells/mm^2 postoperatively. The 2014 study by Wade et al. [65] also reported good improvement of astigmatism from 4.57 ± 2.05 D preoperatively (topographic) to 1.58 ± 1.25 D postoperatively (refractive), with 76.2% of eyes within 1 D of predicted manifest astigmatism at the last visit (mean follow-up of 14.7 months). UDVA and CDVA ≥20/30 were reported in 67% (14/21 eyes) and 81% (17/21 eyes) of cases, respectively.

Conclusion

In summary, there are currently several treatment options for post-PK astigmatism. Incisional surgery has been investigated in several older series. It has shown moderate effectiveness in cylinder reduction but proved to be unpredictable. Currently, incisional surgery can be used to prime the cornea before laser correction is applied. Laser ablation with PRK or LASEK has been proven to be equally effective in terms of the correction of refraction. A common complication like haze can be diminished by applying MMC to the cornea after laser ablation. Refractive results with LASIK seem to be similar to those with surface ablation. Long-term studies on LASIK show good effectiveness for the correction of refractive errors, but

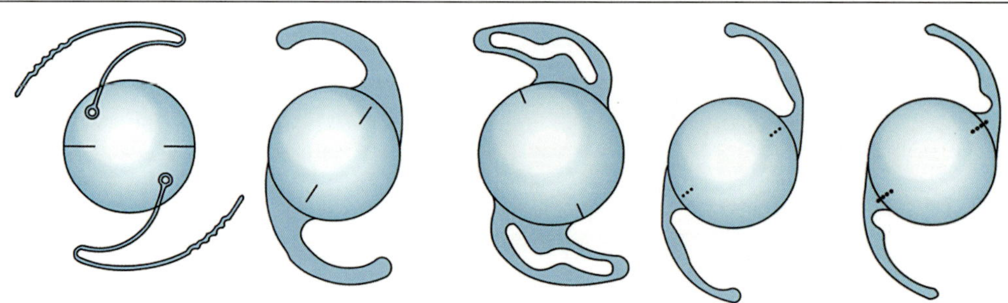

Company	HumanOptics	Oculentis	Rayner	Alcon	AMO
Type	MicroSil	Lentis Tplus	T-flex	Acrysof T3-T9	Tecnis
Material	Silicon optic, PMMA haptics	Hydrophilic acrylic, hydrophobic surface	Hydrophilic acrylic	Hydrophobic acrylic	Acrylic
Spherical range	−3.0 to +31.0 D	0 to +30.0 D	−10.0 to +35.0 D	+6.0 to +30.0 D	+5.0 to +34.0 D
Cylinder range	+2.0 to +12.0 D	+0.5 to +12.0 D	+1.0 to +11.0 D	+1.5 to +6.0 D	+1.0 to +4.0 D
Cylinder steps	1.0 D	0.75/0.01 D	0.25 D	0.75 D	0.5 to 1.0 D
Incision	3.4 mm	2.6 mm	<2.0 mm	2.2 mm	?
Toricity	Monotoric back	Monotoric front	Monotoric front	Monotoric back	Monotoric front
Aspheric	No	Yes	Yes	Yes	Yes
Remarks	Custom-made	Custom-made, plate and loop model	Custom-made	–	–

AMO = Abbott Medical Optics Inc.; PMMA = poly(methyl methacrylate).

flap complications can occur. There is no consensus on the refractive effect of a sole flap cut. The implantation of phakic or pseudophakic toric IOLs can generate excellent refractive results, but both techniques require some preoperative thought. Phakic toric IOLs cause more endothelial cell loss in post-PK patients than in patients with virgin eyes, and this cell loss can eventually result in re-PK if corneal decompensation occurs. Fortunately, phakic toric IOLs can be removed without much difficulty. In patients scheduled for pseudophakic toric IOL implantation, it is very important to consider if re-PK is likely to occur in the future. If so, introducing a pIOL on top of the implanted monofocal pseudophakic IOL might be a more preferable option.

References

1 Karabatsas CH, Cook SD, Sparrow JM: Proposed classification for topographic patterns seen after penetrating keratoplasty. Br J Ophthalmol 1999;83:403–409.

2 Brooks SE, Johnson D, Fischer N: Anisometropia and binocularity. Ophthalmology 1996;103:1139–43.

3 van Rij G, Cornell FM, Waring GO 3rd, et al: Postoperative astigmatism after central vs eccentric penetrating keratoplasties. Am J Ophthalmol 1985;99:317–320.

4 Kerenyi A, Suveges I: Corneal topographic results after eccentric, biconvex penetrating keratoplasty. J Cataract Refract Surg 2003;29:752–756.

5 Eggink FA, Nuijts RM: A new technique for rigid gas permeable contact lens fitting following penetrating keratoplasty. Acta Ophthalmol Scand 2001;79:245–250.

6 Visser ES, Visser R, van Lier HJ, et al: Modern scleral lenses part I: clinical features. Eye Contact Lens 2007;33:13–20.

7 Geerards AJ, Vreugdenhil W, Khazen A: Incidence of rigid gas-permeable contact lens wear after keratoplasty for keratoconus. Eye Contact Lens 2006;32:207–210.

8 Koay PY, McGhee CN, Crawford GJ: Effect of a standard paired arcuate incision and augmentation sutures on post-keratoplasty astigmatism. J Cataract Refract Surg 2000;26:553–561.

9 Hardten DR, Lindstrom RL: Surgical correction of refractive errors after penetrating keratoplasty. Int Ophthalmol Clin 1997;37:1–35.

10 Wilkins MR, Mehta JS, Larkin DF: Standardized arcuate keratotomy for post-keratoplasty astigmatism. J Cataract Refract Surg 2005;31:297–301.

11 Poole TR, Ficker LA: Astigmatic keratotomy for post-keratoplasty astigmatism. J Cataract Refract Surg 2006;32:1175–1179.

12 Hjortdal JO, Ehlers N: Paired arcuate keratotomy for congenital and post-keratoplasty astigmatism. Acta Ophthalmol Scand 1998;76:138–141.

13 Bochmann F, Schipper I: Correction of post-keratoplasty astigmatism with keratotomies in the host cornea. J Cataract Refract Surg 2006;32:923–928.

14 Geggel HS: Arcuate relaxing incisions guided by corneal topography for post-keratoplasty astigmatism: vector and topographic analysis. Cornea 2006;25:545–557.

15 Hoffart L, Touzeau O, Borderie V, et al: Mechanized astigmatic arcuate keratotomy with the Hanna arcitome for astigmatism after keratoplasty. J Cataract Refract Surg 2007;33:862–868.

16 Fares U, Mokashi AA, Al-Aqaba MA, et al: Management of postkeratoplasty astigmatism by paired arcuate incisions with compression sutures. Br J Ophthalmol 2013;97:438–443.

17 Cleary C, Tang M, Ahmed H, et al: Beveled femtosecond laser astigmatic keratotomy for the treatment of high astigmatism post-penetrating keratoplasty. Cornea 2013;32:54–62.

18 Kumar NL, Kaiserman I, Shehadeh-Mashor R, et al: IntraLase-enabled astigmatic keratotomy for post-keratoplasty astigmatism: on-axis vector analysis. Ophthalmology 2010;117:1228–1235.e1.

19 Nubile M, Carpineto P, Lanzini M, et al: Femtosecond laser arcuate keratotomy for the correction of high astigmatism after keratoplasty. Ophthalmology 2009;116:1083–1092.

20 Hoffart L, Proust H, Matonti F, et al: Correction of postkeratoplasty astigmatism by femtosecond laser compared with mechanized astigmatic keratotomy. Am J Ophthalmol 2009;147:779–787.e1.

21 Ghanem RC, Azar DT: Femtosecond-laser arcuate wedge-shaped resection to correct high residual astigmatism after penetrating keratoplasty. J Cataract Refract Surg 2006;32:1415–1419.

22 Lisa C, Garcia-Fernandez M, Madrid-Costa D, et al: Femtosecond laser-assisted intrastromal corneal ring segment implantation for high astigmatism correction after penetrating keratoplasty. J Cataract Refract Surg 2013;39:1660–1667.

23 Campos M, Hertzog L, Garbus J, et al: Photorefractive keratectomy for severe postkeratoplasty astigmatism. Am J Ophthalmol 1992;114:429–436.

24 Lazzaro DR, Haight DH, Belmont SC, et al: Excimer laser keratectomy for astigmatism occurring after penetrating keratoplasty. Ophthalmology 1996;103:458–464.

25 Amm M, Duncker GI, Schroder E: Excimer laser correction of high astigmatism after keratoplasty. J Cataract Refract Surg 1996;22:313–317.

26 Tuunanen TH, Ruusuvaara PJ, Uusitalo RJ, et al: Photoastigmatic keratectomy for correction of astigmatism in corneal grafts. Cornea 1997;16:48–53.

27 Bansal AK: Photoastigmatic refractive keratectomy for correction of astigmatism after keratoplasty. J Refract Surg 1999;15(2 suppl):S243–S245.

28 Bilgihan K, Ozdek SC, Akata F, et al: Photorefractive keratectomy for post-penetrating keratoplasty myopia and astigmatism. J Cataract Refract Surg 2000;26:1590–1595.

29 Hjortdal JO, Ehlers N: Treatment of post-keratoplasty astigmatism by topography supported customized laser ablation. Acta Ophthalmol Scand 2001;79:376–380.

30 Leccisotti A: Photorefractive keratectomy with mitomycin C after deep anterior lamellar keratoplasty for keratoconus. Cornea 2008;27:417–420.

31 Huang PY, Huang PT, Astle WF, et al: Laser-assisted subepithelial keratectomy and photorefractive keratectomy for post-penetrating keratoplasty myopia and astigmatism in adults. J Cataract Refract Surg 2011;37:335–340.

32 Rajan MS, O'Brart DP, Patel P, et al: Topography-guided customized laser-assisted subepithelial keratectomy for the treatment of postkeratoplasty astigmatism. J Cataract Refract Surg 2006;32:949–957.

33 Chang DH, Hardten DR: Refractive surgery after corneal transplantation. Curr Opin Ophthalmol 2005;16:251–255.

34 Donnenfeld ED, Kornstein HS, Amin A, et al: Laser in situ keratomileusis for correction of myopia and astigmatism after penetrating keratoplasty. Ophthalmology 1999;106:1966–1974; discussion 1974–1975.

35 Rashad KM: Laser in situ keratomileusis for correction of high astigmatism after penetrating keratoplasty. J Refract Surg 2000;16:701–710.

36 Kwitko S, Marinho DR, Rymer S, et al: Laser in situ keratomileusis after penetrating keratoplasty. J Cataract Refract Surg 2001;27:374–379.

37 Malecha MA, Holland EJ: Correction of myopia and astigmatism after penetrating keratoplasty with laser in situ keratomileusis. Cornea 2002;21:564–569.

38 Barraquer CC, Rodriguez-Barraquer T: Five-year results of laser in-situ keratomileusis (LASIK) after penetrating keratoplasty. Cornea 2004;23:243–248.

39 Buzard K, Febbraro JL, Fundingsland BR: Laser in situ keratomileusis for the correction of residual ametropia after penetrating keratoplasty. J Cataract Refract Surg 2004;30:1006–1013.

40 Hardten DR, Chittcharus A, Lindstrom RL: Long term analysis of LASIK for the correction of refractive errors after penetrating keratoplasty. Cornea 2004;23:479–489.

41 Webber SK, Lawless MA, Sutton GL, et al: LASIK for post penetrating keratoplasty astigmatism and myopia. Br J Ophthalmol 1999;83:1013–1018.

42 Busin M, Arffa RC, Zambianchi L, et al: Effect of hinged lamellar keratotomy on postkeratoplasty eyes. Ophthalmology 2001;108:1845–1851; discussion 1851–1852.

43 Alio JL, Javaloy J, Osman AA, et al: Laser in situ keratomileusis to correct post-keratoplasty astigmatism; 1-step versus 2-step procedure. J Cataract Refract Surg 2004;30:2303–2310.

44 Kollias AN, Schaumberger MM, Kreutzer TC, et al: Two-step LASIK after penetrating keratoplasty. Clin Ophthalmol 2009;3:581–586.

45 Nuijts RM, Abhilakh Missier KA, Nabar VA, et al: Artisan toric lens implantation for correction of postkeratoplasty astigmatism. Ophthalmology 2004;111:1086–1094.

46 Moshirfar M, Barsam CA, Parker JW: Implantation of an Artisan phakic intra-ocular lens for the correction of high myopia after penetrating keratoplasty. J Cataract Refract Surg 2004;30:1578–1581.

47 Moshirfar M, Feilmeier MR, Kang PC: Implantation of verisyse phakic intra-ocular lens to correct myopic refractive error after penetrating keratoplasty in pseudophakic eyes. Cornea 2006;25:107–111.

48 Tahzib NG, Cheng YY, Nuijts RM: Three-year follow-up analysis of Artisan toric lens implantation for correction of postkeratoplasty ametropia in phakic and pseudophakic eyes. Ophthalmology 2006;113:976–984.

49 Bourne WM, Nelson LR, Hodge DO: Central corneal endothelial cell changes over a ten-year period. Invest Ophthalmol Vis Sci 1997;38:779–782.

50 Bourne WM, Hodge DO, Nelson LR: Corneal endothelium five years after transplantation. Am J Ophthalmol 1994;118:185–196.

51 Ing JJ, Ing HH, Nelson LR, et al: Ten-year postoperative results of penetrating keratoplasty. Ophthalmology 1998;105:1855–1865.

52 Doors M, Berendschot TT, Webers CA, et al: Model to predict endothelial cell loss after iris-fixated phakic intraocular lens implantation. Invest Ophthalmol Vis Sci 2010;51:811–815.

53 Doors M, Tahzib NG, Eggink FA, et al: Use of anterior segment optical coher-ence tomography to study corneal changes after collagen cross-linking. Am J Ophthalmol 2009;148:844–851.e2.

54 Baumeister M, Buhren J, Kohnen T: Po-sition of angle-supported, iris-fixated, and ciliary sulcus-implanted myopic phakic intraocular lenses evaluated by Scheimpflug photography. Am J Ophthalmol 2004;138:723–731.

55 Baikoff G: Anterior segment OCT and phakic intraocular lenses: a perspective. J Cataract Refract Surg 2006;32:1827–1835.

56 Baikoff G, Bourgeon G, Jodai HJ, et al: Pigment dispersion and Artisan phakic intraocular lenses: crystalline lens rise as a safety criterion. J Cataract Refract Surg 2005;31:674–680.

57 Guell JL, Morral M, Gris O, et al: Evalua-tion of Verisyse and Artiflex phakic in-traocular lenses during accommodation using Visante optical coherence tomog-raphy. J Cataract Refract Surg 2007;33:1398–1404.

58 Alfonso JF, Lisa C, Abdelhamid A, et al: Posterior chamber phakic intraocular lenses after penetrating keratoplasty. J Cataract Refract Surg 2009;35:1166–1173.

59 Koivula A, Zetterstrom C: Phakic intra-ocular lens for the correction of hypero-pia. J Cataract Refract Surg 2009;35:248–255.

60 McMullan TF, Goldsmith C, Illingworth CD: Toric posterior chamber (in-the-bag) intraocular lens implantation to correct postpenetrating keratoplasty astigmatism. Eye (Lond) 2007;21:150–152.

61 de Sanctis U, Eandi C, Grignolo F: Phacoemulsification and customized toric intraocular lens implantation in eyes with cataract and high astigmatism after penetrating keratoplasty. J Cataract Refract Surg 2011;37:781–785.

62 Buchwald HJ, Lang GK: [Cataract sur-gery with implantation of toric silicone lenses for severe astigmatism after kera-toplasty]. Klin Monbl Augenheilkd 2004;221:489–494.

63 Kersey JP, O'Donnell A, Illingworth CD: Cataract surgery with toric intraocular lenses can optimize uncorrected postop-erative visual acuity in patients with marked corneal astigmatism. Cornea 2007;26:133–135.

64 Viestenz A, Kuchle M, Seitz B, et al: [To-ric intraocular lenses for correction of persistent corneal astigmatism after penetrating keratoplasty]. Ophthalmo-loge 2005;102:148–152.

65 Wade M, Steinert RF, Garg S, et al: Re-sults of toric intraocular lenses for post-penetrating keratoplasty astigmatism. Ophthalmology 2014;121:771–777.

66 Bahar I, Levinger E, Kaiserman I, Sansanayudh W, Rootman DS: IntraLase-enabled astigmatic keratoto-my for postkeratoplasty astigmatism. Am J Ophthalmol 2008;146:897–904.

Rudy M.M.A. Nuijts, MD, PhD
University Eye Clinic Maastricht, Maastricht University Medical Center
P. Debyelaan 25
NL–6202 AZ, Maastricht (The Netherlands)
E-Mail rudy.nuijts@mumc.nl

Güell JL (ed): Cornea. ESASO Course Series. Basel, Karger, 2015, vol 6, pp 39–53
DOI: 10.1159/000381491

Femtosecond Laser-Assisted Penetrating and Lamellar Keratoplasty

Leonardo Mastropasqua · Mario Nubile

Ophthalmology Clinic, Centre of Excellence in Ophthalmology, National High-Tech Eye Center (CNAT), University 'G. d'Annunzio' of Chieti-Pescara, Chieti, Italy

Abstract

The continuous evolution of corneal transplantation has recently demonstrated that the surgical approach based on selective lamellar keratoplasty represents the gold standard for the treatment of corneal disease. The replacement of the diseased corneal layers via anterior lamellar or endothelial keratoplasty clearly gives advantages to patients in terms of safety and outcomes. However, the classical method of penetrating keratoplasty has also recently undergone evolution and refinements. The introduction of femtosecond laser technology to clinical practice, after its wide use for refractive surgical corneal procedures, allowed for a significant refinement in terms of precision and customization of both penetrating and lamellar keratoplasty. The main advantages of using femtosecond lasers are represented by the possibility of performing complex-shaped trephination in both the donor and recipient tissues (for example, top-hat or zig-zag cut profiles) and the great precision of lamellar dissection. However, cut quality and interface smoothness still represent critical points to be improved.

Introduction

A new era in the field of high-precision corneal microsurgery started in the beginning of this century with the introduction of femtosecond laser (FSL) technology in clinical practice. FSL uses the physical principle of photodisruption in order to achieve an effect; that is, a nonthermal ablation process induced using light in the infrared range produces cavitation gas bubbles. The pulse duration is in the sub-picosecond range and produces spots that are only a few microns wide. Cuts require precisely and accurately generating a sequence of adjacent bubbles. The precision of this laser permits various types of corneal stromal cuts with customizable shape, depth, dimension and orientation [1, 2].

Numerous FSL systems that are currently available for corneal surgical procedures include the Abbott Medical Optics FSLs (IntraLase and iFS, Abbott Medical Optics, Santa Ana, Calif., USA), the VisuMax (Carl Zeiss Meditec, Jena,

Germany), the Femto LDV (Ziemer Ophthalmic Systems Group, Port, Switzerland), and the VICTUS (Bausch and Lomb/Technolas Perfect Vision GmBH, Munich, Germany). These systems present important differences in terms of technical specifications and the specific methods implemented for imaging and operating on the eye, such as pulse frequency (ranging from 80 to 1,000 kHz), pulse duration, energy delivered per single pulse, bubble spatial separation, geometrical construction and distribution of spots in order to create a resection, type of laser contact with the corneal surface (patient docking: applanation or curved interface), and type of corneal resections [3, 4]. However, in general, they achieve similar effects on the corneal tissue by delivering multiple laser pulses with a duration of several femtoseconds at a predetermined depth and location within the cornea that cleave the tissue along a plane.

The aim of this chapter is not to provide a comprehensive description of FSL-based corneal graft surgery presently available for specialists for whom specific textbooks and publications are available [5]. The principal aim is to present a brief overview of the main applications of FSL in keratoplasty that in the recent years has promoted a significant evolution in the field of corneal surgery. These advances have driven the industry towards continuous research and development in order to improve the systems and have favored subsequent FSL-based surgery of the crystalline lens.

Theoretically, FSL is capable of producing any kind of wound configuration with precise control of all dimensions with a degree of precision that is not possible with manual techniques. Currently, FSL-based techniques are used for the most part in refractive surgery for making anterior corneal flaps in laser-assisted in situ keratomileusis (LASIK) [6–8], for implantation of intrastromal corneal ring segments [9], for intrastromal refractive lenticule extraction [10] and, recently, in the field of corneal transplantation to generate custom-shaped corneal trephination profiles in penetrating keratoplasty (PK) [11–13] and deep corneal dissection in lamellar keratoplasty [14]. Additionally, FSLs have been used to create arcuate incisions to correct high astigmatism in post-keratoplasty corneas [15, 16]. FSL systems have been used to create trephinations and dissections both in donor and recipient tissue in PK, anterior lamellar keratoplasty (ALK) and Descemet membrane stripping endothelial keratoplasty. In the following paragraphs, a brief description of these applications is presented.

Principles of Femtosecond Laser Stromal Dissections

The femtosecond ray is also defined as intrastromal because it targets the corneal stroma on a specific plane of focus, leaving the corneal tissue it crosses intact. This is due to its mechanism of action: the given wavelength of the infrared laser beam dissects tissue via a process called photodisruption [1, 2, 5]. If solid matter is transparent, like the cornea, the laser beam will simply pass through it. The extreme brevity of FSL pulses allows a very high number of photons to be delivered to the target point during an extremely short time period. When the density of photons is high, enough multiple photons are likely to hit the bound electrons in a short period of time. When the number of photons hitting a specific point in space is sufficiently high to supply the energy necessary to liberate electrons from the atoms, tissue vaporization is initiated. However, the energy of each individual laser pulse remains low enough to ensure that collateral damage to the surrounding tissue is minimized [5].

The laser is focused on a spot diameter of less than 2–3 microns at the desired depth in the corneal stroma with an optical system that is finely controlled by the computer. The beam must pass through the overlying corneal layers to reach the plane of focus, bringing thousands of pulses within a short temporal sequence. The location of

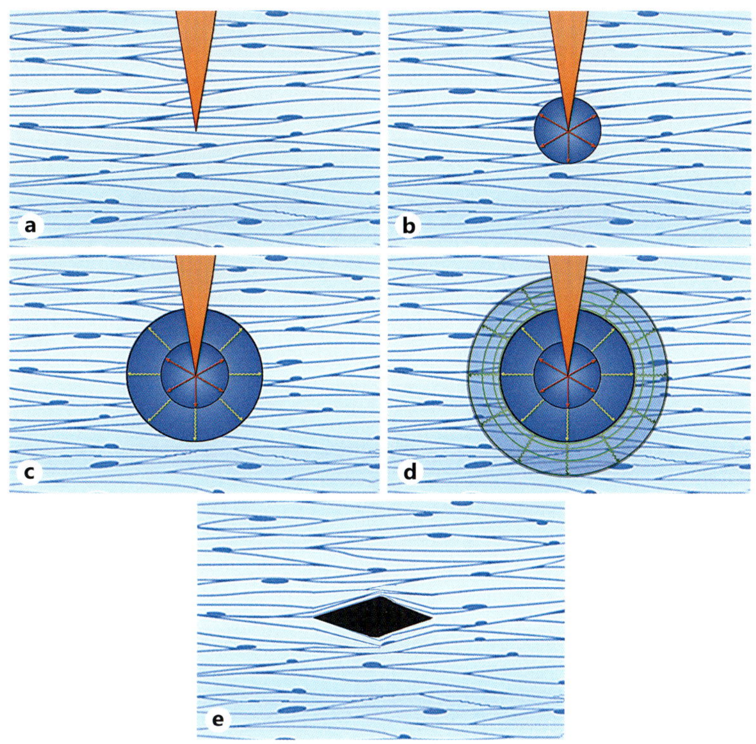

Fig. 1. a Each femtosecond laser (FSL) beam is focused at the desired depth of the corneal stroma. **b** The laser-matter interaction produces a bubble of vaporized matter called 'plasma' (orange arrows). **c** A fast increase in temperature and pressure within the bubble plasma causes volume expansion at supersonic speed (yellow arrows). **d** Reducing the speed of expansion due to tissue interaction produces shock-waves that propagate into the surrounding tissue. **e** A focal dissection of the stroma is then created. Thousands of adjacent cavitation bubbles produce dissection planes of the desired size, depth and orientation. (Modified from [5].)

each of the target spots is programmed in order to create a precise predefined geometrical pattern. Thus, it is possible to create a dissection, tunnel, cut or combinations of these with a high degree of precision and repeatability.

The intrastromal FSL received Food and Drug Administration approval in December 1999 and was presented for the first time during the annual meeting of the American Academy of Ophthalmology in October 2000.

Figure 1 outlines the steps of corneal femtodissection. When the laser beam is focused at a certain depth within the cornea, it initiates a process of multiphoton ionization of corneal tissue and creates a small microplasma bubble of the vaporized corneal tissue [5]. The size of the microplasma bubble varies from less than 1 micron to 5 microns in diameter, depending on the pulse energy. Microplasma contains water and carbon dioxide. As the gas within the microplasma rapidly expands, it becomes a cavitation bubble. Depending on the laser pulse energy, the diameter of the cavitation bubble may be several times larger than the initial microplasma bubble. The individual cavitation bubbies either coalesce or are very close to each other, with only thin bridges of tissue separating them. As the process continues and the cavitation bubbies implode, the water and carbon dioxide are absorbed via endothelial cell pump action. Any remaining bridges can then be broken with a spatula during the flap lift in the LASIK procedure (fig. 2) or during their insertion into the laser-generated channels in intracorneal ring segments or with a dissecting instrument during donor and recipient button removal in keratoplasty.

To reduce tissue bridges and to facilitate tissue separation, the distance between the laser pulses can be decreased. The pulses can, in fact, be placed so closely together that the oncoming pulse

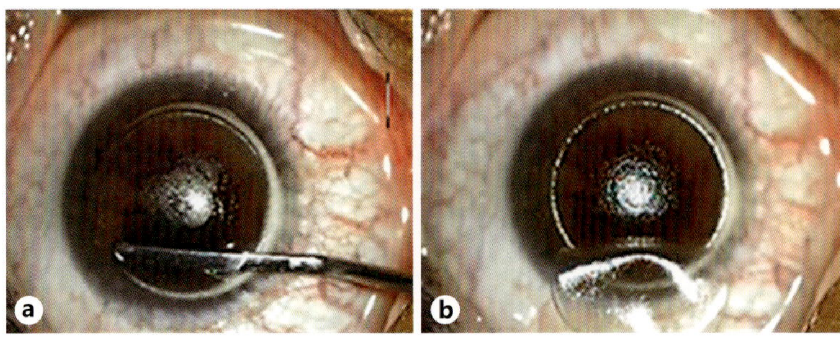

Fig. 2. After a stromal dissection plane is created by the FSL (a laser-assisted in situ keratomileusis flap in this case), a blunt instrument is inserted into the interface through the side cut and is used to separate the residual tissue bridges to lift the flap.

overlaps the collapsed cavitation bubble created by the previously applied pulse. The positioning of the spots can be programmed and executed with a degree of accuracy and precision that allows complex 3D cut patterns to be made.

Femtosecond Laser-Assisted Penetrating Keratoplasty

PK is by far the most common corneal transplant surgery that has been performed in the world in the last century. It requires the replacement of the entire thickness of the cornea with a diameter ranging from 3 to 5 mm (PK tectonic) to very large diameters when the peripheral cornea is affected. Generally, in the classical indications for PK-optic procedures (keratoconus, bullous keratopathy, leucomas, etc.), the diameter is between 7.50 and 8.50 mm in order to reduce the risk of transplant rejection and to control the excessive induction of astigmatism. The circular trephination of the cornea is based on mechanical trephines with sharp knives of varying diameter.

The technique of PK has reached a high level of standardization, especially in recent decades, and even now, PK is the most common technique used in corneal transplant surgery in Europe and throughout the world. In the last decade, however, a radical change in surgical techniques has caused an exponential increase in the number of lamellar grafts (front and endothelial cells). It is expected that the lamellar-selective techniques

(mainly lamellar keratoplasty for anterior corneal diseases with healthy endothelium such as keratoconus, dystrophies, leucomas and posterior lamellar endothelial keratoplasty for pathologies only affecting the endothelium) will progressively replace PK, leaving only a small portion of patients in whom it is not possible to perform selective techniques or under circumstances of urgency, infection or perforation. Among the various fields of corneal surgery that use FSL, techniques of PK were among the first proposed, experimentally studied, and subsequently implemented clinically. In fact, the ability to create complex 3D geometrical patterns is the main theoretical advantage of this technology compared to conventional trephination.

Shaped Penetrating Keratoplasty. Complex Profiles of Femtosecond Laser Trephinations Complex Sagittal Trephination Profiles Nonmechanical trephination PK using FSLs has recently been reported [11–13]. The advantages are the precision of the cut and the potential for custom-shaped corneal trephination (fig. 3), such as 'top-hat' [11] or 'zig-zag' [12] profiles that, at least theoretically, lead to a more precise matching of donor-recipient wound edges and impart a greater mechanical stability of the graft.

FSLs can make linear or complex geometrical trephination cuts, thus increasing the strength and the integrity of the donor-recipient interface (fig. 3). The complex geometric profiles include the following: 'top-hat' (with a wider anterior di-

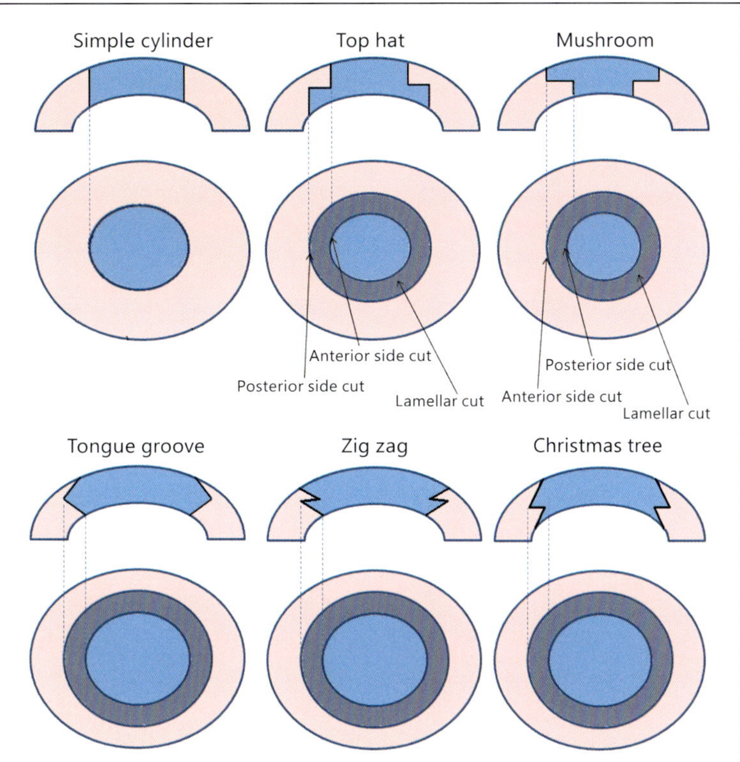

Fig. 3. Schematic representation of complex FSL trephination shapes for penetrating keratoplasty (PK). Top left panel, classical mechanical blade-based vertical trephination. The other panels show cross-section and en-face representations of different FSL cut shapes for PK. Note that the anterior and posterior side cut length, position and orientation as well as the size and depth of the interconnecting lamellar cut can be varied according to the surgeon's choice and the patient's corneal characteristics.

ameter), 'mushroom' (with an even greater outer diameter), 'tongue -groove', 'zig-zag' and 'Christmas tree'. Note that the 'mushroom' profile may be useful under conditions such as keratoconus due to the large refractive front surface of the button, while the 'top-hat' profile can provide benefits to corneal endothelium diseases since it results in the replacement of a greater number of endothelial cells. Recent studies showed that among different forms of trephination analyzed for the treatment of sclerocorneal rings in the human artificial anterior chamber, the biomechanical properties (clinically observed as resistance to trauma, postoperative dehiscence and leakage) were better in those types of profiles with respect to the standard types [17, 18]. Complex configurations of the trephination provide better matching at the wound edge between the donor and the recipient. The new reference profile that showed

the best sealing biomechanics was the 'top hat' profile. It has been observed that the 'top hat' configuration in PK is associated with less wound leakage and provides the structural advantage of looser sutures, which, theoretically, may decrease suture-induced astigmatism and may allow for faster visual recovery.

A recent clinical trial comparing the outcomes of 'mushroom' FSL-enabled keratoplasty with those of conventional PK in eyes with keratoconus reported that the former resulted in less astigmatism and a trend toward higher endothelial cell counts than conventional PK, along with similar postoperative best-corrected visual acuity [19]. Similarly, incisions using zig-zag femtosecond trephination in patients with keratoconus showed faster visual recovery and better long-term outcomes than those using mechanical trephines for PK [20].

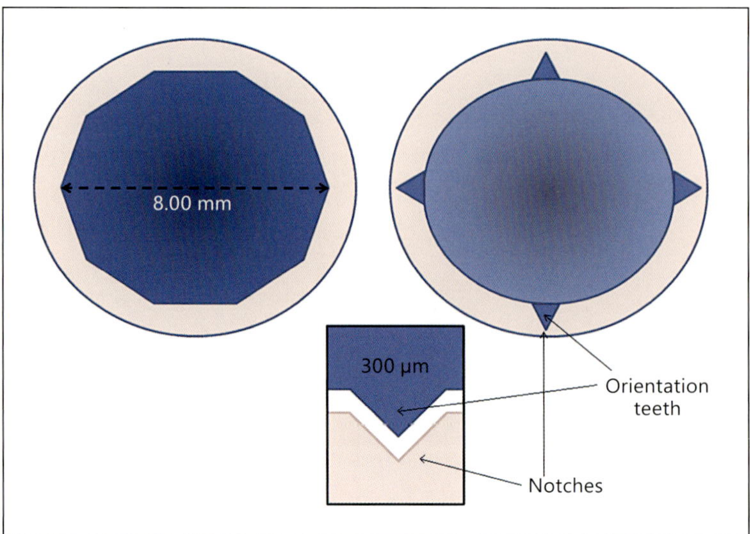

Fig. 4. Schematic representation of complex FSL trephination shapes for PK: **a** 'decagonal' profile; **b** 'orientation teeth and notches' profile. **c** Insert showing the size and the junction type of the graft.

In conclusion, FSL-assisted PK provides good visual outcomes, at least comparable to conventional technique, offering early visual rehabilitation due to precise graft-host alignment and reduced astigmatism in the early postoperative months.

Complex En-Face Trephination Profiles
The feasibility of creating orientation teeth in the graft (also called 'positional spikes') and corresponding notches in the trephination profile of PK that act as 'key in a keyhole' coupling has been shown [13]. Another reported option is to create angle-shaped trephination profiles with 'decagonal keratoplasty' [21]. The aim of these modifications is to improve the fitting of the donor button into the recipient cornea, thus increasing the rotational stability of the graft (fig. 4, 5).

A different type of trephination complex geometry is based on linear cuts associated with a modified classic circular shape. These geometries are based on profiles in which the anterior-posterior direction (epithelium and endothelial lines) appears to be linear, while the overall shape of the cut is not simply circular. Among the various proposals that have been applied clinically are those based on the technique of interlocking triangular teeth embedded in the circular profile (orientation teeth and notches) and decagonal trephination (polygonal rather than circular). In these profiles, the contact surface between donor-recipient surfaces is not increased by increasing the intra-stromal contact angle of the surfaces but rather results from a profile with linear joints linked to the corners or irregular shapes in the linear profile (fig. 4). The decagonal keratoplasty profile was accomplished with a 40 kHz FSL (fig. 4) using the same diameter of 8.0 mm on the donor and recipient with a cutting angle of 90° and using a mixed suture with 10 sutures on the corners of the decagon and a continuous 10 steps on the sides [21]. The polygonal PK permits an accurate positioning of the flap and easier suturing of the flap to recipient bed, reducing rotational button slippage. The potential advantages of this new pattern compared to the round PK could include faster visual recovery and reduced induced astigmatism [21].

PK with a complex profile called orientation teeth and notch was also implemented using the same diameter (8.0 mm) for the donor and the recipient and using 90° cuts (fig. 4, 5). This profile

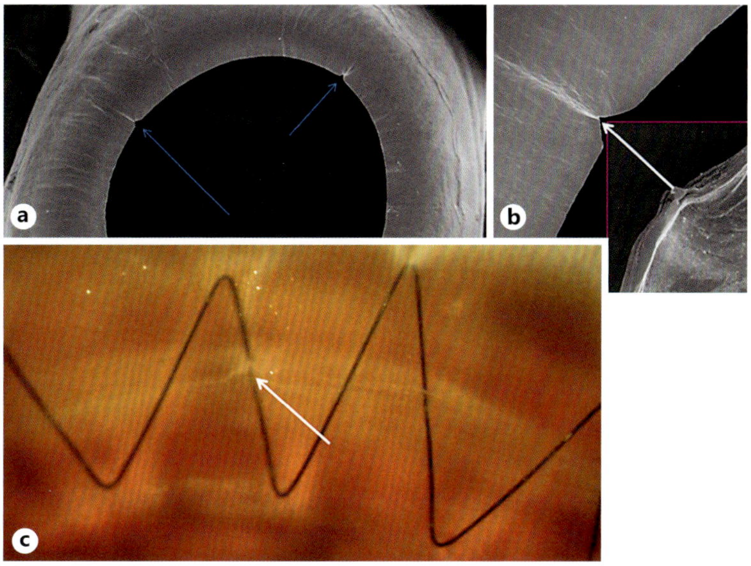

Fig. 5. FSL-assisted 'orientation teeth' profile for PK. **a** Orientation notches are visible on the presented scanning electron microscopy (SEM) image of the sclerocorneal rim of the donor tissue. **b** SEM image illustrating the orientation teeth and notch fitting. **c** Detailed postoperative image of a PK in which the suture track passes through a positional spike, indicated by the arrow.

reduces torsional slippage during suturing and, thus, postoperative surgically induced astigmatism [13].

It is worth noting that complex profiles of any type are closely linked to the efficacy of the cuts and the correct functioning of the laser. An incomplete cut, a less-than-perfect diameter or an irregular profile would represent a greater intraoperative surgical problem than that which would be encountered during a mechanical circular trephination. Therefore, the quality of the FSL cut is a fundamental factor for complex profiles. Later in this chapter, we will describe the characteristics and the evolution of PK trephination from a histological prospective.

Simple Angled Femtosecond Laser Trephination Profiles

Another option is the use of straight cuts for trephination profiles but with an angled orientation with respect to the corneal surface, as opposed to mechanical trephination that is always vertical. These profiles could offer some advantages in terms of greater wound strength, increased contact area between the donor and host

tissues and reduced endothelial area to be transplanted while maintaining a sufficiently large outer diameter (as shown in fig. 6).

The FSL has been used clinically also to perform simple linear trephination [22]. However, by changing the angle of trephination, it is possible to perform PK with an oblique cut edge that provides a greater surface area of contact between the donor and recipient tissues. For example, it is possible to perform a full-thickness trephination with a variable angle from the epithelium to the endothelium. With a classic mechanical trephination (analogous to what occurs during the preparation of the donor button with the punch), the epithelial line-endothelium direction, which has an inclination of about 65° with respect to the tangent to the corneal surface and, therefore, is parallel to the antero-posterior axis of the bulb, is followed (fig. 7a). The FSL can be used to perform variable angles of trephination. The most convenient angles are those greater than 65°, generally between 90° and 120° (fig. 7b). In this case, the diameter of the epithelial flap is greater than the endothelial diameter proportionally to the chosen inclination angle. For example, with a 90°

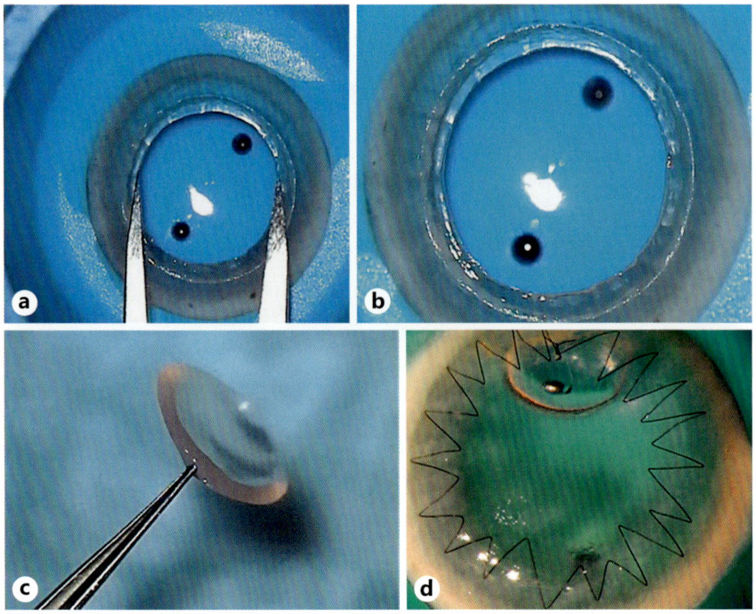

Fig. 6. FSL-assisted trephination with an angled profile (120° in this case). **a** and **b** After FSL-assisted trephination, the inner diameter was 7.25 mm, and the outer (epithelial) diameter was 9.00 mm (25% more epithelium than endothelium). **c** The trephined corneal button was removed and positioned to show the angled profile of the trephination. **d** The artificial anterior chamber after the graft is sutured in place.

angle trephination, if an endothelial diameter of 7.1 mm is chosen, an epithelial diameter of 8.2 mm will be obtained. For an angle of 120° (fig. 6), an endothelial surface diameter of 6.75 mm corresponds to a superficial diameter of 8.75 mm. This imparts some theoretical advantages compared to traditional vertical cuts: the diameter of endothelium and, consequently, the endothelial antigen load are smaller (remember that the cell density (cells/area) for a given number of endothelium cells decreases in proportion to r^2). Even with the same endothelial diameter, the superficial diameter is greater and is therefore closer to the limbus, thus minimizing induced astigmatism. The linear surface of the donor-recipient contact is greater thanks to the oblique surface, thus improving the seal. The angled profile also reduces the risk of leakage, since a sort of interlocking funnel is produced. A shallower and less tense suture can be applied, thus reducing the compression of the periphery of the transplant, respecting the physiological curvature of the entire flap and the anterior chamber space (fig. 7). It should be emphasized, however, that there is no

scientific evidence supporting the hypothesis that reducing the diameter of endothelial PK is associated with a proportional reduction of the risk of rejection. Antigen sensitization always occurs first on the surface of antigen-presenting cells.

Histological Findings of Femtosecond Laser Cut Quality

The cut quality that can be obtained with FSLs is influenced by numerous factors that are either laser-dependent or tissue-dependent. The most important factors among the former are the frequency and the energy of the laser impulses, the spacing of the spots, and the geometric profile. The latter factors include depth, the interlacing and the cross-angles between the collagen lamellae, tissue opacity (edema, leucoma and vascularization) and the spatial orientation of the cuts (fig. 8a, b).

Over the years, the overall attainable quality of cuts has been constantly improving thanks to the increase in pulse frequency and the progressive reduction of the energy applied to form each spot (fig. 8c, d).

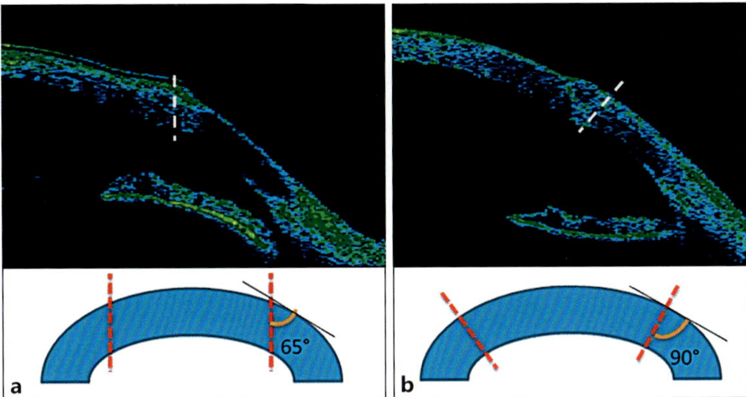

Fig. 7. A traditional penetrating transplant in an early postoperative phase on optical coherence tomography (OCT) of the anterior segment (left). Below is a diagram of the trephination 'vertical' to 65° degrees. The donor-recipient interface is indicated by a dashed white line. The donor and recipient interface is vertical, and the suture reduces the curvature of the peripheral cornea and 'crushes' the anterior chamber. A PK with FSL trephination (right) with a linear geometry of 90°. The cut is angled, which is also visible on OCT. The passage of the suture includes approximately 60% of the corneal thickness. This technique is associated with a better curvature of the cornea and to a more physiological geometry of the anterior chamber.

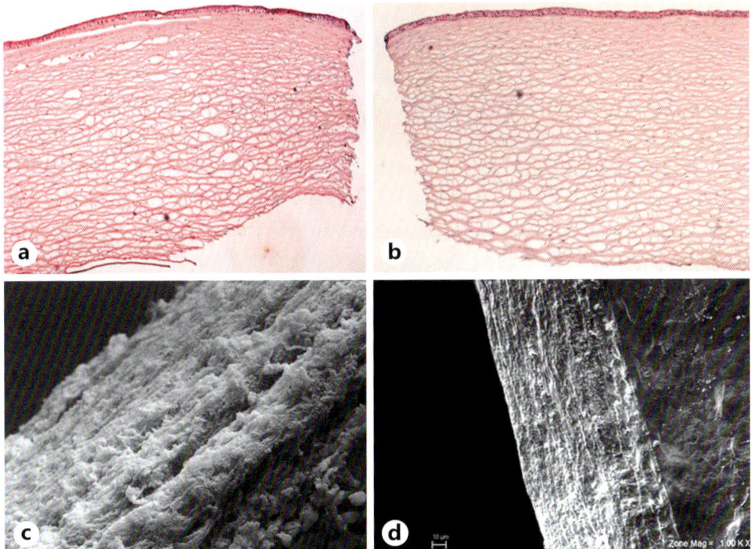

Fig. 8. Histological technique for analyzing the quality of the corneal cut obtained with FSL using full-thickness transparency. **a** Hematoxylin-eosin staining after a vertical cut was performed on an edematous cornea with the laser operating at 40 kHz. Edema is confirmed by the increased interlamellar stromal spaces and the detached stromal epithelium. In this case, the cut quality was not optimal, and some frayed and irregular fibrils can be seen on the margin. **b** Hematoxylin-eosin staining after a similar treatment in a nonedematous cornea. The better cut quality is seen with a clean surface. **c** SEM after a perforating cut for PK performed with a FSL at 40 kHz. Small irregularities with frayed fibrils can be seen on the cut surface. **d** SEM after a 500 kHz FSL cut. The cut surface does not present the same irregularities.

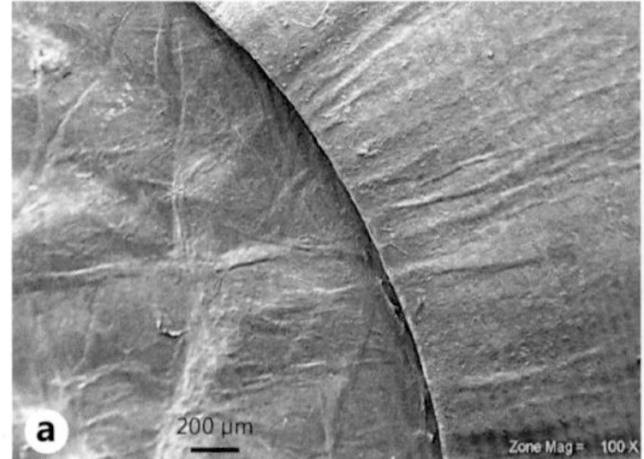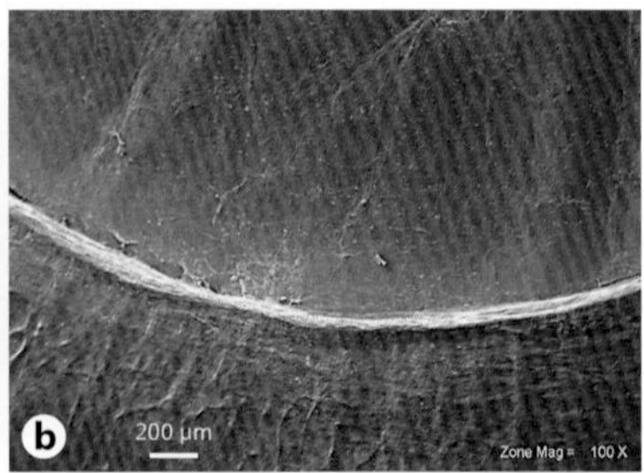

Fig. 9. Differences in lamellar dissection quality due to the frequency (and the energy) of different FSL systems. SEM image showing the stromal surface after a lamellar dissection using a FSL at 60 kHz (left) or at a greater frequency (500 kHz) and lower energy levels per spot (right). The FSL cuts showed better surface quality even at greater depths in the rear stroma.

Vertical cuts, or cuts that are not parallel to the horizontal plane of the corneal lamellae, interrupt the integrity of the fibers at a more or less perpendicular plane. This results in a relatively simple separation of the cut margins, and the eventual presence of residual fibrils do not represent a clinically relevant problem because their presence only influences the healing of the transplant border, not the optic zone. It is necessary, however, especially when using complex geometric patterns, that the cut surfaces be consistent and easily separated in order to avoid any macroscopic tissue fraying that could result in a nonoptimal fit between the donor and recipient tissues. On the other hand, when performing a deep stromal dissection that is parallel to the plane of the fibers (such as in deep anterior and posterior lamellar keratoplasty) with an FSL, the cutting quality of the laser is greatly influenced by the tissue parameters and the depth. These aspects will be further discussed in the chapters dedicated to lamellar keratoplasty techniques.

Femtosecond Laser-Assisted Lamellar Keratoplasty

ALK has the advantages of reducing intraoperative complications, enabling faster visual rehabilitation, and decreasing the risk of graft rejection. Posterior lamellar keratoplasty (endothelial keratoplasty) offers the advantages of avoiding wound-dehiscence risk, suture-related problems and astigmatism while reducing the rejection rate following PK. The use of FSL in these procedures combines the advantages of selective lamellar keratoplasty with the surgical precision of laser surgery. FSL-assisted lamellar keratoplasty techniques include FSL-assisted ALK (FSL-ALK), FSL-assisted deep ALK, and FSL-assisted endothelial keratoplasty [23].

Initially, the possibility of creating a deep lamellar dissection of the cornea led to the use of an FSL system for anterior (ALK) and posterior lamellar keratoplasty (Descemet membrane stripping automatic endothelial keratoplasty (DSAEK)) [23–25]. The aim of these procedures in the field of ALK or deep ALK was to create both donor and recipient trephination and lamellar cuts with perfect shapes and customized profiles (similar to PK). The first FSL systems used were characterized by high energy levels and relatively low frequency (less than 60 kHz). One of the main problems encountered when using these systems, particularly when cutting the deep corneal stroma, is irregular stromal and uneven surfaces (stucco-like appearance). This problem may be related to the FSL-energy dispersion and attenuation that occur when cutting through the rear deep stroma with laser systems that were optimized to create LASIK flaps in the anterior corneal layers, characterized by a looser fibrillar configuration and a greater water content with respect to the anterior stroma. This concept is illustrated in figure 9.

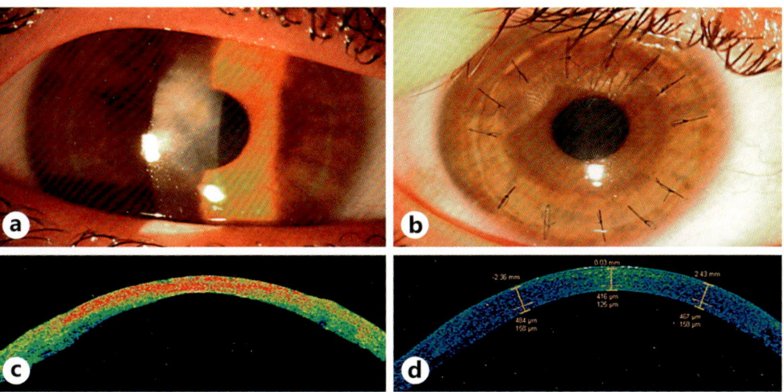

Fig. 10. a Preoperative slit lamp photograph of a case of postinfectious stromal scar that was a candidate for FSL-assisted ALK (FSL-ALK). **b** Postoperative appearance of the same case 4 months after FSL-ALK and selective suture removal to control astigmatism. **c** Preoperative anterior segment OCT image showing central corneal thinning. **d** Postoperative OCT image showing the deep lamellar interface (125 µm above the endothelium in the center) and the restoration of a normal corneal thickness.

FSL systems have been successfully used to perform ALK in clinical practice (fig. 10). The advantages of these systems are the relative ease with which they perform the dissection on the recipient, yielding extreme precision in terms of diameter, depth and side-cut pattern. Similarly, the donor dissection can be prepared by mounting the donor sclerocorneal rim on an artificial anterior chamber. Perfect shapes and sizes of the graft can be obtained. Surgeons can customize the thickness of the lamellar dissection, even with differences between the donor and recipient thicknesses. This 'mismatch' can be useful in cases of preoperative corneas presenting with significant thinning (i.e., after postinfectious scarring, as shown in fig. 10). A greater thickness of the donor dissection compared with the recipient dissection can restore a normal corneal thickness after surgery.

The main disadvantage of the FSL-ALK procedure is easily seen when treating keratoconic corneas with irregular thinning. All FSL systems produce a lamellar cut parallel to the epithelial surface, thus reproducing the irregularity in the residual stromal bed of the donor. This leads to poor outcomes, mainly due to the postoperative irregular geometry of the graft. In addition, to date, the interface quality and, therefore, the visual results obtainable with FSL-ALK are not comparable to the outcomes of manual techniques in which Descemet's membrane (DM) is exposed. Therefore, FSL-ALK should be preferably indicated in cases of anterior stromal scars or stromal corneal dystrophies with healthy endothelium. The main advantages of performing such procedures is the fact that surgery to remove the pathological stroma can usually be performed under local (often topical) anesthesia, leaving a relatively smooth stromal interface with perfect matching of the donor and recipient lamellar button profiles (fig. 11).

Recently, shaped trephination profiles have also been used to create a better match between the donor button and the recipient stromal bed in FSL-ALK and deep ALK, with the advantages of better mechanical stability and improved healing of stepped corneal wounds [26–29].

Similarly, FSLs have been utilized to create the lamellar dissection in the donor cornea for posterior lamellar keratoplasty lenticule preparation (FSL-assisted DSAEK) as an alternative to microkeratomes [30].

Nowadays, DSAEK represents the most utilized transplant technique for the treatment of corneal endothelial dysfunction leading to corneal edema and consequent vision loss, such as Fuchs' endothelial dystrophy and pseudophakic

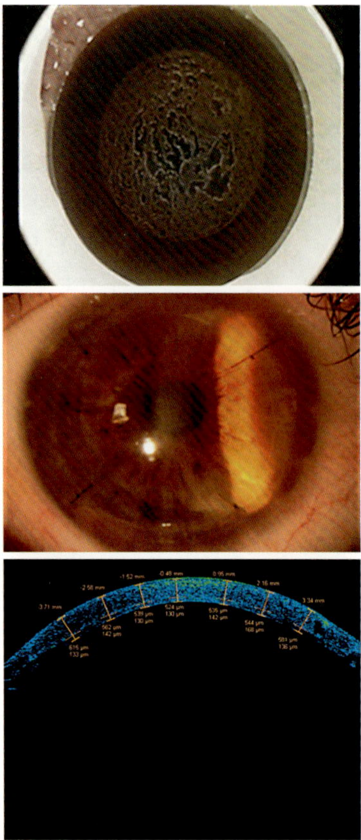

Fig. 11. FSL-ALK. Top panel, the intraoperative view of the FSL during the lamellar dissection phase in the recipient eye. Note that the procedure in this case was performed under topical anesthesia, facilitated by a firm suction onto the surface of the eye. The middle panel shows the postoperative appearance of an FSL-ALK case with only 4 single sutures left in place. The bottom panel presents the postoperative OCT image in which the deep and regular lamellar interfaces are clearly visible.

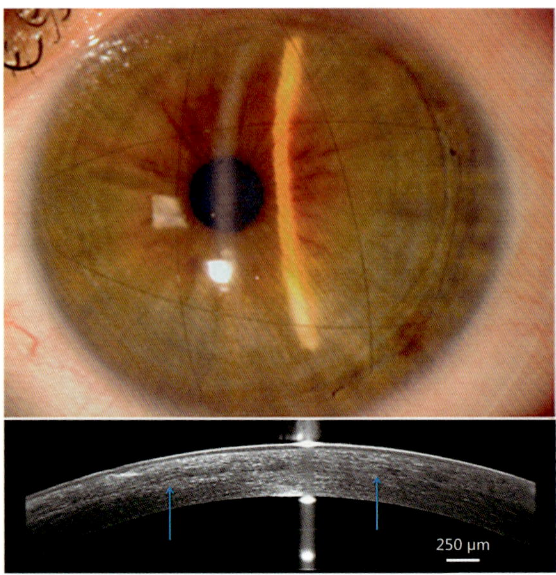

Fig. 12. FSL-ALK performed for a post-PRK stromal scar. Top panel, the postoperative slit-lamp image 1 week after surgery. Only `bridge' superficial surface sutures held the 9.0 mm graft in place. Bottom panel, the high-resolution OCT image illustrates the mid-stromal interface, with a mild amount of stromal edema.

bullous keratopathy. In this procedure, the pathological DM and the endothelium are usually stripped off, and a thin lamella of donor cornea containing the endothelium, the DM and a variable portion of rear stroma is inserted into the anterior chamber of the recipient eye and is fixed in place by the aid of an air bubble. Generally, the posterior lamellar disc is prepared using a micro-keratome. Alternatively, an FSL is used to dissect the donor tissue at the desired depth (fig. 12), which is established based on the pre-cut pachymetry of the donor cornea. This option could be particularly useful for the preparation of very thin DSAEK grafts (as shown in fig. 13 and 14).

If complex angled trephination profiles are used, fewer sutures can be applied in order to reduce suture-related problems or induced astigmatism, as shown in figures 11 and 15, respectively. Also, sutureless FSL-ALK has been proposed by different authors [25]. However, we recommend the use of at least containment sutures to be left in place for the first few months in order to avoid possible spontaneous or trauma-induced button dislocation (fig. 12).

The main advantages of preparing the posterior lamellar disc for DSAEK using the FSL are

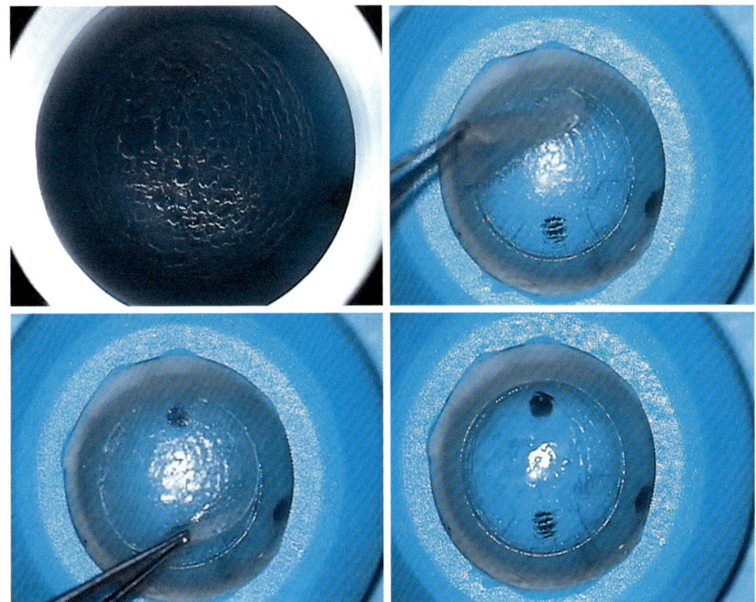

Fig. 13. Sequence of intraoperative images illustrating the preparation of the Descemet stripping endothelial keratoplasty posterior lamellar disc using the FSL (500 kHz in this case). Top left panel, the FSL is used to perform the deep lamellar dissection (400 microns) and the vertical trephination cut, while the sclerocorneal donor rim is mounted to the artificial anterior chamber. Bottom left and top right panels, the anterior lamellar disc was removed. Bottom right panel, the posterior lamella was ready for punching.

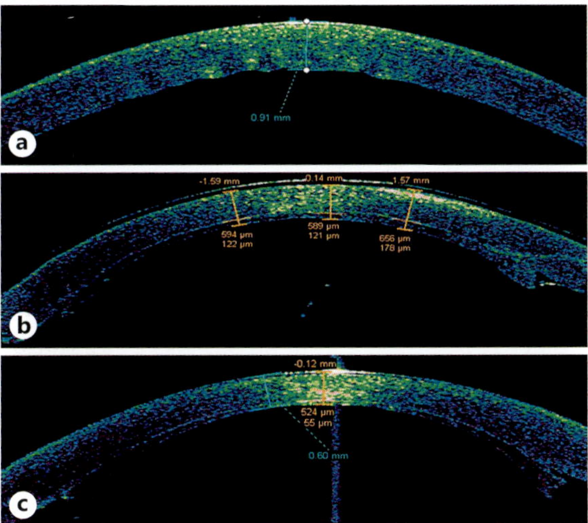

14

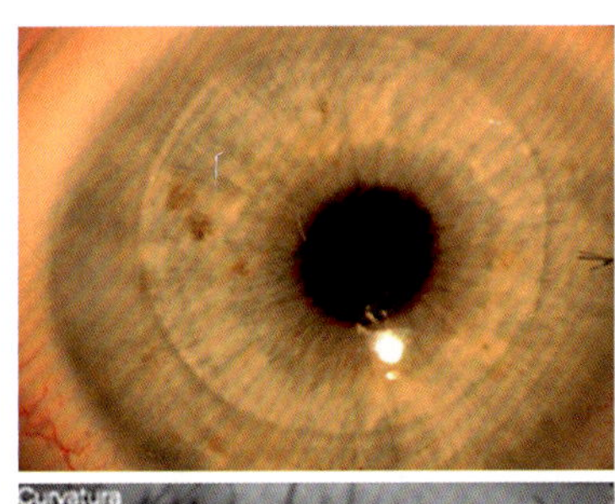

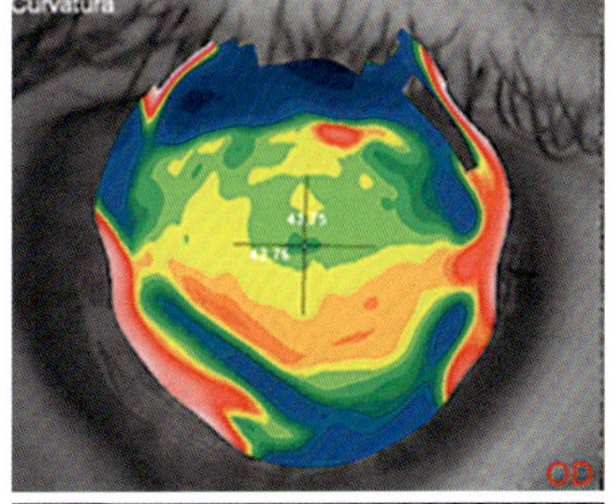

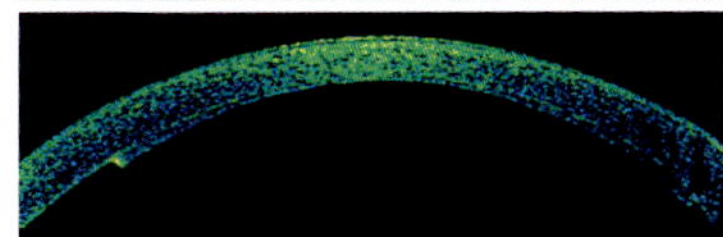

15

Fig. 14. An example of FSL-assisted ultra-thin Descemet membrane stripping automatic endothelial keratoplasty imaged with anterior segment OCT. **a** Edematous donor cornea. **b** Postoperative appearance of the same case 1 week after surgery showing a central graft thickness of approximately 120 microns. **c** After complete resolution of swelling, 1 month after surgery, the central thickness of the graft had reduced to less than 60 microns.

Fig. 15. An example of the clinical outcome after FSL-assisted Descemet membrane stripping automatic endothelial keratoplasty. Top panel, slit-lamp postoperative image showing a clear cornea and a transparent interface. Middle panel, regular corneal topography with no astigmatism. Bottom panel, anterior segment OCT image showing a thin, regular posterior graft.

represented by the possibility of optimizing the thickness and the shape of the donor button, theoretically favoring a better postoperative peripheral profile (fig. 14) of the graft and a consequent refractive shift. However, the quality of the interface attained by the FSL-assisted posterior stromal dissection may critically affect visual outcomes; therefore, microkeratome-assisted DSAEK still represents the gold standard technique [24, 31].

Laser technologies are continuously and rapidly evolving; therefore, a progressive increase in their applications in the field of corneal grafting and the improvement of clinical outcomes will probably represent the basis for the spread of such automated procedures in the near future.

References

1 Sugar A: Ultrafast (femtosecond) laser refractive surgery. Curr Opin Ophthalmol 2002;13:246–249.
2 Farid M, Steinert RF: Femtosecond laser-assisted corneal surgery. Curr Opin Ophthalmol 2010;21:288–292.
3 Lubatschowski H: Overview of commercially available femtosecond lasers in refractive surgery. J Refract Surg 2008; 24:102–107.
4 Binder PS, Sarayba M, Ignacio T, et al: Characterization of submicrojoule femtosecond laser corneal tissue dissection. J Cataract Refract Surg 2008;34:146–152.
5 Faktorovic EG: Femtodynamics. A Guide to Laser Settings and Procedure Techniques to Optimize Outcomes with Femtosecond Lasers. Thorofare, NJ, SLACK Incorporated, 2009.
6 Netto MV, Mohan RR, Medeiros FW, et al: Femtosecond laser and microkeratome corneal flaps: comparison of stromal wound healing and inflammation. J Refract Surg 2007;23:667–676.
7 Patel SV, Maguire LJ, McLaren JW, et al: Femtosecond laser versus mechanical microkeratome for LASIK: a randomized controlled study. Ophthalmology 2007;114:1482–1490.
8 Salomao MQ, Wilson SE: Femtosecond laser in laser in situ keratomileusis. J Cataract Refract Surg 2010;36:1024–1032.
9 Shabayek MH, Alió JL: Intrastromal corneal ring segment implantation by femtosecond laser for keratoconus correction. Ophthalmology 2007;114:1643–1652.
10 Sekundo W, Kunert K, Russman C, et al: First efficacy and safety study of femtosecond lenticule extraction for the correction of myopia: six months results. J Cataract Refract Surg 2008;34:1513–1520.
11 Price FW Jr, Price MO: Femtosecond laser shaped penetrating keratoplasty: one-year results utilizing a top-hat configuration. Am J Ophthalmol 2008;145:210–214.
12 Farid M, Kim M, Steinert RF: Results of penetrating keratoplasty performed with a femtosecond laser zigzag incision initial report. Ophthalmology 2007;114:2208–2212.
13 Mastropasqua L, Nubile M, Lanzini M, et al: Orientation teeth in non-mechanical femtosecond laser corneal trephination for penetrating keratoplasty. Am J Ophthalmol 2008;146:46–49.
14 Yoo SH, Kymionis GD, Koreishi A, et al: Femtosecond laser-assisted sutureless anterior lamellar keratoplasty. Ophthalmology 2008;115:1303–1307.e1.
15 Nubile M, Carpineto P, Lanzini M, et al: Femtosecond laser arcuate keratotomy for the correction of high astigmatism after keratoplasty. Ophthalmology 2009; 116:1083–1092.
16 Kumar NL, Kaiserman I, Shehadeh-Mashor R, et al: IntraLase-enabled astigmatic keratotomy for post-keratoplasty astigmatism: on-axis vector analysis. Ophthalmology 2010;117:1228–1235.
17 Maier P, Böhringer D, Birnbaum F, et al: Improved wound stability of top-hat profiled femtosecond laser-assisted penetrating keratoplasty in vitro. Cornea 2012;31:963–966.
18 Malta JB, Soong HK, Shtein R, et al: Femtosecond laser-assisted keratoplasty: laboratory studies in eye bank eyes. Curr Eye Res 2009;34:18–25.
19 Levinger E, Trivizki O, Levinger S, et al: Outcome of 'mushroom' pattern femtosecond laser-assisted keratoplasty versus conventional penetrating keratoplasty in patients with keratoconus. Cornea 2014;33:481–485.
20 Gaster RN, Dumitrascu O, Rabinowitz YS: Penetrating keratoplasty using femtosecond laser-enabled keratoplasty with zig-zag incisions versus a mechanical trephine in patients with keratoconus. Br J Ophthalmol 2012;96:1195–1199.
21 Proust H, Baeteman C, Matonti F, et al: Femtosecond laser-assisted decagonal penetrating keratoplasty. Am J Ophthalmol 2011;151:29–34.
22 Por YM, Cheng JY, Parthasarathy A, et al: Outcomes of femtosecond laser-assisted penetrating keratoplasty. Am J Ophthalmol 2008;145:772–774.
23 Yoo SH, Hurmeric V: Femtosecond laser-assisted keratoplasty. Am J Ophthalmol 2011;151:189–191.
24 Cheng YY, Schouten JS, Tahzib NG, et al: Efficacy and safety of femtosecond laser-assisted corneal endothelial keratoplasty: a randomized multicenter clinical trial. Transplantation 2009;88:1294–1302.
25 Yoo SH, Kymionis GD, Koreishi A, et al: Femtosecond laser-assisted sutureless anterior lamellar keratoplasty. Ophthalmology 2008;115:1303–1307.
26 Chan CC, Ritenour RJ, Kumar NL, et al: Femtosecond laser-assisted mushroom configuration deep anterior lamellar keratoplasty. Cornea 2010;29:290–295.

27 Shehadeh-Mashor R, Chan CC, Bahar I, et al: Comparison between femtosecond laser mushroom configuration and manual trephine straight-edge configuration deep anterior lamellar keratoplasty. Br J Ophthalmol 2014;98:35–39.

28 Shehadeh-Mashor R, Chan C, Yeung SN, et al: Long-term outcomes of femtosecond laser-assisted mushroom configuration deep anterior lamellar keratoplasty. Cornea 2013;32:390–395.

29 Price FW Jr, Price MO, Grandin JC, et al: Deep anterior lamellar keratoplasty with femtosecond-laser zigzag incisions. J Cataract Refract Surg 2009;35:804–808.

30 Soong HK, Mian S, Abbasi O, et al: Femtosecond laser-assisted posterior lamellar keratoplasty: initial studies of surgical technique in eye bank eyes. Ophthalmology 2005;112:44–49.

31 Cheng YY, van den Berg TJ, Schouten JS, et al: Quality of vision after femtosecond laser-assisted descemet stripping endothelial keratoplasty and penetrating keratoplasty: a randomized, multicenter clinical trial. Am J Ophthalmol 2011; 152:556–566.

Leonardo Mastropasqua
Ophthalmology Clinic, Centre of Excellence in Ophthalmology
National High-Tech Eye Center (CNAT), University 'G. d'Annunzio' of Chieti-Pescara
Via dei Vestini
IT–66100 Chieti (Italy)
E-Mail mastropa@unich.it

Güell JL (ed): Cornea. ESASO Course Series. Basel, Karger, 2015, vol 6, pp 54–65
DOI: 10.1159/000381492

Corneal Collagen Crosslinking Techniques: Updates

Myriam Cassagne · Safa El Hout · François Malecaze

Department of Ophthalmology, Purpan Hospital, Toulouse, France

Abstract

Corneal collagen crosslinking (CXL) is usually practiced on keratoconic corneas to strengthen the corneal biomechanical structure. The conventional CXL procedure, with riboflavin and ultraviolet A (UVA), initially involves corneal de-epithelialization to allow riboflavin penetration into the stroma. Discomfort and complications are related to this corneal debridement. Thus, transepithelial CXL has emerged to substitute for the conventional method. This technique preserves the epithelium and tends to ensure the same efficiency of corneal stiffening. To allow riboflavin penetration through the epithelial barrier, several chemical modifications to riboflavin, such as addition of enhancers (EDTA, benzalkonium chloride or 20% alcohol), and osmolar modifications have been applied. The most studied transepithelial riboflavin is Ricrolin TE®, which combines two enhancers: amino alcohol and EDTA. The results of clinical studies have not demonstrated effectiveness yet. Moreover, the iontophoresis technique, a noninvasive procedure during which a low-intensity electric current is applied to enhance the penetration of riboflavin into the stroma, stands out as being as efficient as conventional application of riboflavin, based on a pre-clinical study. Another area of improvement of CXL is modification of the UVA irradiation profile or shortening of the UVA irradiation time while increasing the irradiation power. A longer follow-up and more investigations are still necessary to define the future of transepithelial CXL, but it is an exciting and rapidly evolving area.

Introduction

Ectatic diseases such as keratoconus or iatrogenic ectasia after laser-assisted in situ keratomileusis (LASIK) are characterized by modification of the cornea's biomechanical properties. Comparison between the biomechanical characteristics of normal and keratoconus corneas reveals alteration of the biomechanical characteristics of the ectatic cornea, precisely in the collagen scaffold and in bonding between collagen molecules [1]. Induction of crosslinks, i.e., formation of chemical bridges between molecules, is an established method in chemistry to increase the elastic modulus of materials. This method is common in odontology: crosslinking of dentinal collagen is practiced in order to enhance the biodegradation resistance and strength of dentin or resin [2]. Crosslinking is a well-regulated physiological process in various connective tissues of the human body (skin, vessels, ocular lens, and cornea) [3, 4]. This process corresponds to protein glycation that increases with aging and in pathological states such as diabetes mellitus and that rigidifies the tissue. This is why patients suffering from diabetes mellitus tend not to show corneal ectasia progression [5].

Corneal collagen crosslinking (CXL) with riboflavin and ultraviolet A (UVA), initially introduced by Seiler et al. in 2003, has emerged as an efficient method for keratoconus treatment [6]. CXL stands out because it is currently the only curative treatment capable of slowing and even halting the evolution of keratoconus by increasing the corneal stiffness [7].

However, CXL may have many adverse effects, mainly related to de-epithelialization during this procedure. Consequently, a new technique that preserves the epithelium while maintaining the same efficiency of corneal stabilization is the main future treatment prospect for progressive keratoconus. Over the last few years, the conventional CXL (C-CXL) technique has undergone various attempts at improvement.

Biomechanics of the Cornea

The biomechanical properties of the cornea are mainly attributable to the stroma since the latter represents 90% of the thickness. The stroma's principal components are collagen molecules, which are assembled into long, uniform-diameter fibrils (31–34 nm) organized into stabilized fibers called lamellae (1–2 µm thickness and 100–200 µm width) [8].

The fibrils reach their specific firmness due to physiological crosslinks between collagen molecules. CXL is enzymatically regulated by the lysyl oxidase, which catalyzes the amino groups of amino acids (such as lysine) into aldehyde groups [9]. These aldehyde groups create covalent bridges either between each other or with other amino acids within one or different fibrils. For keratoconus patients, defects have been observed within the lysyl oxidase-coding gene [10]. A high pH level in tears also induces alteration of lysyl oxidase activity. Some studies show a decrease in protease inhibitor levels, generating higher digestive activity [11].

The spatial arrangement of the corneal fibers is another major factor that influences the biomechanical properties and the shape of the cornea. This arrangement has been deeply investigated, thanks to several studies and a large variety of imaging modalities (e.g., electron microscopy, x-ray diffraction, confocal microscopy, nonlinear optical imaging techniques) [1, 12–17].

The basic model described by Meek et al. is based upon a vertical parallel stack of collagen lamellae in 200 successive planes, with every plane oriented along a reference vector rotated about 90° relative to its neighbor [1, 18]. More recently, x-ray scattering studies of corneal collagen orientation showed the heterogeneous organization of the collagen fibers across the cornea; the organization of the fibers into orthogonal sheets in the central cornea contrasts with the tangential orientation of the fibers in the periphery [19]. The peripheral lamellae seem to follow the corneal circumference. A study by Daxer et al. on collagen fiber orientation showed that two thirds of the stromal fibers in the normal cornea are within a 45° sector around the horizontal and vertical meridians, whereas the remaining one third is oriented in the oblique sectors [1, 8]. Many studies revealed that the orthogonal arrangement is altered in keratoconus corneas, especially inside the apical scar [14, 20]. This structural disorganization may explain the stiffness loosening that induces corneal bugling and stromal thinning.

Furthermore, three-dimensional evaluation of the corneal collagen ultra-structure by Winkler et al. using nonlinear optical imaging techniques such as second harmonic-generated imaging led to a model of fiber organization including complex intertwining between collagen fibers from

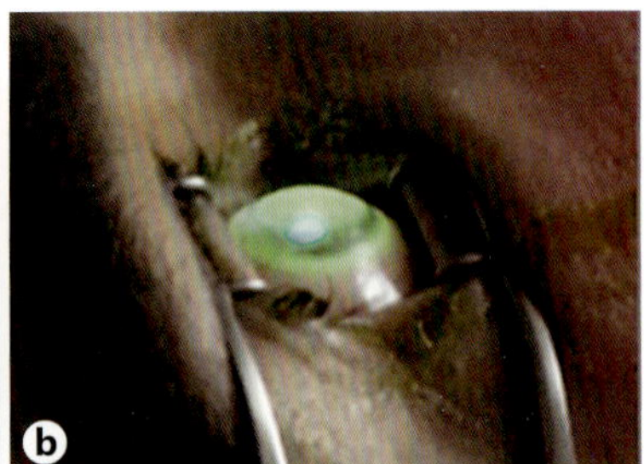

Fig. 1. Conventional corneal collagen crosslinking procedure. Riboflavin instillation on de-epithelialized cornea (**a**) followed by ultraviolet A irradiation (**b**).

different layers and three-dimensional fiber branching [16]. Moreover, the cornea was subdivided into three layers (anterior, middle and posterior) using a femtosecond surgical laser. Measurements of the fiber branching density in each of the 3 layers showed that the anterior third is significantly more intertwined than the middle and posterior thirds are. Mechanical testing of each layer showed a significant increase in the effective elastic modulus of the third (anterior) layer compared to the two others.

Thus, the elastic modulus increases with branching density, and consequently, biomechanical properties depend upon the collagen fiber interconnectivity. This feature is most important in the third (anterior) layer of cornea, thus making it the target of CXL.

Biochemical Principles of Conventional Corneal Collagen Crosslinking

The aim of CXL with riboflavin and UVA is to accelerate the physiological mechanism of protein glycation. How CXL actually works is controversial, but it is thought that CXL creates bonds between collagen molecules in order to rigidify the anterior corneal stroma [21, 22]. UVA light acts as catalyzer. Riboflavin (vitamin B_2) acts as photosensitizer that absorbs energy from UVA light and that is then excited, leading to the production of covalent bonds between amino groups either within the collagen molecules or between proteo-glycan core proteins and collagen. Riboflavin and UVA crosslink type I collagen α and β chains into larger polymers and also crosslink major proteoglycan core proteins (keratocan, lumican, mimecan, and decorin) into higher-molecular-weight polymers. In addition, crosslinks are formed between collagen and proteoglycan core proteins depending on the core protein [23]. This reaction requires oxygen molecules and generates oxygen free radicals by riboflavin photolysis [24].

Another potential ex vivo mechanism of CXL is an increase in the production of fibronectin and tissue transglutaminase (an enzyme that crosslinks extracellular matrix proteins) in human keratocytes treated by CXL [25].

Conventional Corneal Collagen Crosslinking

The Conventional Procedure

CXL is performed as an outpatient service on a day-surgery basis. For the current C-CXL treatment method, the corneal stroma is soaked in a riboflavin solution before being exposed to UVA irradiation. Since riboflavin cannot penetrate epithelial cell tight junctions to permeate the corneal stroma, the central corneal epithelium must be debrided across a diameter of 8.0 mm.

The conventional procedure (fig. 1), according to Dresden's protocol [26], requires using an operating block for around 75 minutes. After topical anesthesia, muco-cutaneous disinfection, and application of the lid speculum, the first step is mechanical central de-epithelialization of the cornea over a diameter of 8–9 mm. The second step is stromal saturation by instilling a riboflavin drop every minute over a 30-minute duration (fig. 1a). The last step is central irradiation of the de-epithelialized area using UVA light (wavelength of 365 nm) with an irradiance of 3 mW/cm^2 for 30 minutes (fig. 1b). The patient is asked to focus on the central light-emitting diode of the UVA device. Saturating the anterior segment with riboflavin blocks the transmission of irradiation to posterior intraocular structures [27]. Topical antibiotic therapy is instilled at the end of the intervention, and a therapeutic lens may be placed for about 48 hours.

Efficiency

Several clinical trials highlighted the efficiency and safety of this procedure for progressive keratoconus treatment [28]. Increased stiffness while maintaining corneal transparence has been demonstrated ex vivo with CXL [29]. The resistance to enzymatic degradation is also increased [30]. The sustainability of the results has not yet been demonstrated due to physiological renewal of corneal collagen molecules only every 2–3 years. Because collagen turnover in the stroma is known to take several years, it remains unclear whether the changes in corneal stability reported after CXL will be permanent or whether its effects are temporary. The question of further treatment is then evoked. The long-term effects of standard and modified protocols for CXL should be reviewed thoroughly in studies with longer follow-up. However, in an uncontrolled retrospective study, Raiskup-Wolf et al. showed that the flattening process continues over a period of years, as they followed a large cohort of patients for up to 6 years and reported arrested keratoconus progression [26].

In practice, results have shown that keratoconus progression is stopped in 90% of cases, with a mean decrease of 2D in maximal keratometry readings. In parallel, although it is not the main goal of CXL, significant improvement in the best-corrected visual acuity could be observed [6, 31–37].

The mean failure rate, defined as an increase in the maximal keratometry reading by over one diopter over 1 year, varies between 8 and 10% [30]. No major risk factor for failure has been clearly identified, although some have presented a keratometry value over 58 diopters as a criterion. However, this topic currently remains a matter of controversy.

Adverse Effects

Various studies report a low incidence of side effects or complications, affecting around 3% of cases (1–10%) [38, 39]. These complications are mostly due to epithelium removal, which is indispensable for intrastromal riboflavin penetration, and are listed as follows:

– Pain during the first 48 hours post-surgery due to de-epithelialization [40].
– Temporary decrease in visual acuity during the first 3 months [41].
– Haze-like aspect due to a transitory anterior corneal scar responsible for a reversible decrease in visual acuity within the first 3 months [42].
– Aseptic peripheral infiltrates (due to the immune reaction to staphylococcal antigens) [43].
– Infectious keratitis, with the main identified germs being *Pseudomonas aeruginosa*, *Escherichia coli*, *Staphylococcus epidermidis*, and even plurimicrobial infections [44, 45].
– Herpetic reactivation [46].
– Endothelial decomposition on a thin cornea (<400 μm), as endothelial cells can be damaged starting from 0.35 mW/cm^2 irradiation (the administered dose according to the conventional protocol is 0.18 mW/cm^2).
– Stromal opacities (in around 3% of cases) or permanent haze [41].
– Corneal necrosis [43].

These complications can be severe and may necessitate corneal transplantation.

One must note that the majority of complications are due to de-epithelialization. Thus, a CXL technique that preserves the epithelium would allow avoidance of these complications and undesirable negative effects.

New Corneal Collagen Crosslinking Riboflavin/Ultraviolet A Techniques

Riboflavin Application
Given the above-mentioned complications, a procedure preserving the epithelium while presenting the same efficiency as C-CXL would represent a safer therapy for patients suffering from progressive keratoconus. The standard riboflavin solution is 0.1% concentrated 5-phosphate riboflavin in 10 ml of 20% dextran T500. Its hydrophilic characteristics prevent full diffusion through the lipophilic epithelium. Moreover, electrostatic repulsion between the corneal surface and the riboflavin, which are both negatively charged, limits penetration [47].

When epithelial removal was restricted to a grid pattern of superficial debridement, this was not sufficient to permit homogeneous saturation of the stroma [48].

Prolonging the exposure time did not lead to better saturation in a cornea with intact epithelium [49].

Ensuing attempts consisted of modifying the riboflavin solution formula in order to facilitate its transepithelial penetration. Several enhancers have been proposed to improve riboflavin penetration through the epithelium in the corneal stroma while avoiding epithelial debridement, such as EDTA, benzalkonium chloride or 20% alcohol [50, 51]. Riboflavin in association with anesthetic drops poorly penetrates the cornea [50].

To date, the most studied transepithelial riboflavin is Ricrolin TE® (Sooft, Montegiorgio, FM, Italy), which combines two enhancers: the amino alcohol Tris (trometamol) and EDTA. The results of clinical studies on Ricrolin TE® are contradictory: several have shown some effectiveness, with less pronounced effects than C-CXL, while others have demonstrated ineffectiveness [52, 53]. A recent assessment of the clinical results of transepithelial CXL for patients with progressive keratoconus over a period of 24 months revealed instability of the keratoconus [53]. To date, the efficacy of this treatment is still under investigation, and no prospective randomized clinical study has proven its efficiency.

Raiskup et al. analyzed osmolar modification of riboflavin to enhance its penetration of the epithelium. They found that a transepithelial riboflavin solution should not contain dextran and should contain, 0.01% benzalkonium chloride and 0.44% sodium chloride to promote epithelial permeability by increasing the paracellular conductance [54].

An experimental investigation demonstrated that a riboflavin nanoemulsion (i.e., a submicron-sized oil-in-water emulsion) could be delivered into the stroma of intact epithelium at a similar concentration to that used in the standard technique. A promising method is use of NC-1059, a channel-forming peptide that transiently opens the intact epithelial barrier, thus allowing the penetration of riboflavin. This method apparently has no cytotoxicity [55].

The iontophoresis technique is a noninvasive procedure during which a low-intensity electric current is applied to enhance the penetration of an ionized substance into a tissue. It has been used in various areas of medicine, such as in local anesthetics, transdermal anti-inflammatories or analgesics and transmucosal anti-viral administration [56]. In ophthalmology, the first studies on iontophoresis were performed in the 1940s, with the administration of antibiotics for the treatment of bacterial endophthalmitis and keratitis [57, 58]. Ocular iontophoresis is still being investigated as an answer to the low intraocular bioavailability of drugs in the treatment of several eye disorders of the anterior and posterior segments. This technique has been proposed for the treatment of corneal pathologies such as paecilomyces keratitis [59].

In iontophoresis, the substance is applied via an electrode carrying the same charge as the substance, and a return electrode, which is of the opposite charge, is placed elsewhere in the body to complete the circuit (fig. 2). The substance plays the role of a conductor of current through the tissue. As riboflavin is negatively charged and has a low molecular weight, it is a perfect candidate for the iontophoresis technique, which could allow intrastromal riboflavin diffusion while preserving the corneal epithelium [60]. A pre-clinical study has shown that iontophoresis is as efficient as the conventional application of riboflavin administration and CXL [61]. However, this technique is still under clinical investigation, and long-term studies are necessary to complete the evaluation of iontophoresis.

Moreover, Daxer proposed the direct application of riboflavin to the stroma in one session, without epithelial debridement [62]. This technique combines a new crosslinking method with implantation of a flexible full-ring implant into a corneal pocket. The riboflavin is instilled into the corneal pocket. A case report revealed some favorable results and the safety of this technique [63–65]. The biomechanical effect of CXL using the femtolaser pocket technique is about 50% less pronounced than that after standard CXL. Future studies will show whether the efficacy of the technique can still be improved and whether the clinical effect is sufficient for stabilizing ectatic corneas.

Ultraviolet A Therapy
This therapy is based on the principle of equivalent energy dosing, with the amount of corneal strengthening being energy dependent, and not power dependent. Higher power delivered over a shorter time theoretically provides the same corneal strengthening as the conventional treatment does.

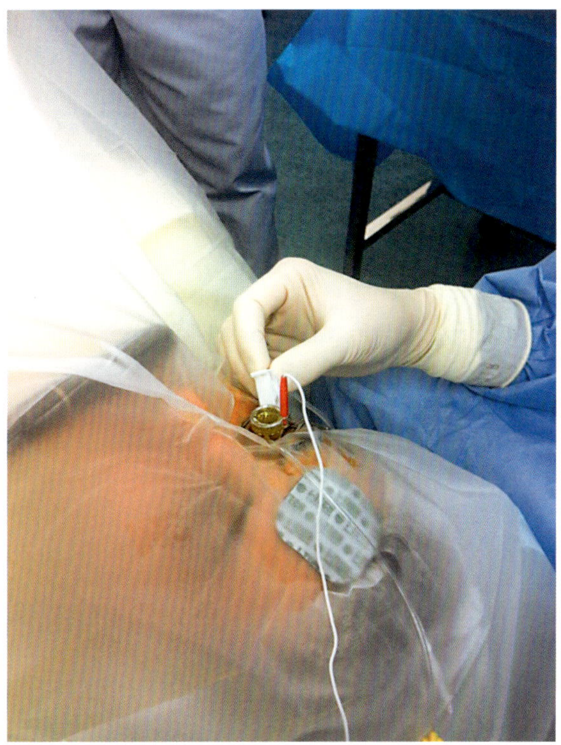

Fig. 2. Riboflavin application by iontophoresis. The main electrode is maintained by a suction ring on the cornea, with intact epithelium. The return electrode is a patch placed on the forehead.

One of the suggested improvements of the CXL procedure is shortening the UVA irradiation time. In fact, the resultant corneal hardening is proportional to the total energy dose delivered to the cornea, and not to the intensity. Hence, equivalent hardening can be generated with C-CXL (30 minutes of irradiation) by increasing the irradiation power in order to apply an equivalent dose of energy to the cornea (according to the Bunsen-Roscoe reciprocity law) [66].

Some competing companies are actually working on this concept. In this framework, the marketed ultraviolet lamp properties are modified in order to deliver 10 mW/cm^2 within 9 minutes instead of 3 mW/cm^2 within 30 minutes. One company is proposing a new device that allows CXL in 3 minutes. Experimental studies have revealed equivalent corneal stiffness between the different approaches, which deliver the same amount of total energy [67, 68].

However, upon a certain threshold value (47 mW/cm^2), the increase in irradiation intensity is no longer associated with the increase in the corneal stiffness. The total energy necessary is 90 mW/cm^2, which corresponds to around 2 minutes of irradiation time [68]. This threshold value for shortening the irradiation duration is explained by the hypothesis that it corresponds to the minimal timeout necessary for oxygen renewal within the stroma. This renewal launches the glycation chemical reaction, which consumes oxygen and produces oxygenated free radicals.

Early clinical studies have revealed the efficiency of 'accelerated' irradiation procedures [68–70]. However, no randomized prospective study has yet proven the noninferiority of UVA-accelerated treatments relative to the conventional procedure. Moreover, the number of samples for these first studies was low, and some of them showed reversible damage of endothelial cells following CXL using an accelerated irradiation approach [68].

Furthermore, modulation of the UVA irradiation profile is a potential prospect for CXL. In fact, the irradiation profile can be adapted to pre-operative inputs (e.g., topography, optical coherence tomography images) of the treated cornea or to fluorescence-based pre-operative procedures to adjust the delivered intensity [71].

Overview of Other Corneal Collagen Crosslinking Procedures

UVA irradiation toxicity and long-term effects on the lens and retina have pushed researchers to explore some new corneal stiffening techniques that avoid UVA use:
– Glutaraldehyde CXL showed a greater increase in corneal rigidity than C-CXL did but exhibited important endothelial toxicity [72].
– Genipin, a natural compound, has been proposed as an alternative CXL method, enhancing the biomechanical properties of the cornea. Similar effects were found with epi-on and epi-off procedures, while cell damage was controlled [73, 74].
– Collagen crosslinking using Bengal rose followed by irradiation with green light has been assessed in rabbit eyes. The first investigations reported attractive results: corneal stiffness was significantly increased by short-term treatment (12 minutes), no kerato-toxicity developed, and the technique could be used on thin corneas (<400 μm) [75].

Clinical Applications

Progressive Keratoconus
Keratoconus is a common bilateral progressive corneal ectatic disease that induces visual impairment by generating irregular astigmatism and paracentral corneal opacities. This disorder typically begins during teenage years; progresses until the age of 30–40 years; and, in severe forms, may necessitate corneal transplantation [76]. Until recently, all keratoconus treatments tended to correct the refractive complications without curing the underlying stromal abnormalities. In contrast, CXL allows arrest of the progression of this disease.

Currently, keratoconus is the main indication for CXL. In keratoconus, the CXL indication always involves disease evolution. This progression can be functional and/or physical and is objectified by topography, followed by a pachymetry or corneal aberrometry study.

However, the problem of progressive keratoconus may arise. In Dresden in 2008, Spoerl et al. suggested that one of the following criteria should be met [26]:

- An increase in the keratometry by >1 diopter over a year.
- A necessity to readapt the contact lens over a 2-year period.
- A loss of visual acuity reported by the patient.

An Italian research team used a more blurred definition within their study, with progression clinically and para-clinically defined over a period of 6 months [33].

An Australian team conducted a comparative study using the following progression criteria over a 1-year period [31]:
- A decrease in the spherical correction by >0.5 diopter.
- A decrease in the cylinder by >1 diopter.
- An increase in the maximal keratometry value by >1 diopter.

In a French study conducted within the 'Centre de Référence National du Kératocône', the progression criteria were as follows [37]:
- An increase in the maximal keratometry reading by >1 diopter over 6 months or by >2 diopters over 1 year.
- A 2-line decrease in the corrected visual acuity over a year.

In fact, the indication for CXL that seems generally agreed upon is based on the presence of the following criteria:
- An increase in the maximal keratometry by more than 1 diopter over a 1-year lead time (or less), established by comparing two successive topographic exams (conducted on the same equipment).
- Conservation of the central corneal transparency.
- Central pachymetry >400 μm.

Ectasia after Laser-Assisted in situ Keratomileusis

Post-LASIK corneal ectasia is one of the most serious side effects of refractive surgery, characterized by progressive thinning of the cornea. CXL using riboflavin and UVA seems to increase the stiffness and biomechanical stability of the cornea [77]. Several studies showed that ectasia post-refractive surgery is successfully treated and even reversed by CXL. In fact, the best-corrected visual acuity was significantly improved, and a considerable effect on flattening and regularizing the corneal curvature was also observed on topography maps after a 12-month follow-up [34, 35, 77, 78].

Pseudophakic Bullous Keratopathy

Many studies seek to evaluate the outcomes of CXL in symptomatic pseudophakic bullous keratopathy with pain and/or a decrease in corneal transparency [79, 80]. Significant improvement and regression of pain scores were noticed during the first 6 months. However, this improvement was shown to be temporary and without long-lasting effects since bullous keratopathy reappeared after a mean of 6 months, with the same symptoms. Consequently, one can deduce that the efficiency of CXL was restrained.

Severe Infectious Keratitis

Moreover, there are indications for CXL for the treatment of severe infectious keratitis and corneal melting [81]. An interventional case series reported positive effects on refractory infectious keratitis not responding to anti-microbial therapy [34, 35, 37]. Martins et al. showed that the riboflavin/UVA combination has anti-microbial efficiency against several bacterial and fungal isolates in vitro [78]. CXL increases stromal resistance against enzymatic digestion and probably allows the destruction of germs in the keratocytes of the anterior stroma [82].

Signs of infection were mostly resolved within 1–2 weeks after the treatment. Despite this fact, some cases still require penetrating keratoplasty due to the state and the extent of scarring [83].

Combined Techniques of Corneal Collagen Crosslinking and Refractive Surgery

Recently, the combined techniques of CXL and refractive corneal surgery have been proposed as a solution to refractive errors in patients with keratectasia. Stiffening the cornea by CXL, along with refractive surgery, could be effective in overcoming refractive abnormalities and biomechanical disorders. Combining CXL with keratorefractive procedures, such as intrastromal corneal ring segment implantation and photorefractive keratectomy, is a promising therapeutic alternative to penetrating keratoplasty or lamellar keratoplasty. In many cases, this combination can improve visual acuity, stabilize ectasia, and delay or even prevent the need for more invasive procedures.

Several promising combinations of CXL and refractive interventions were assessed in different studies:

- Topography-guided photorefractive keratectomy (PRK) followed by CXL [84].
- Intracorneal ring segment implantation with same-day CXL [85–88].
- Intracorneal ring segment implantation followed by sequential same-day topography-guided PRK and CXL with riboflavin and UVA [85, 89, 90].

There is no broad consensus on either the chronology of the procedures (CXL before ring settlement or vice versa) or the timeline for two procedures. However, it seems that CXL should be performed first, followed by another treatment if necessary [91].

Patients who have undergone lamellar keratoplasty for keratoconus have unpredictable, irregular post-operative astigmatism associated with large numbers of higher-order aberrations. Combined treatment with customized excimer laser-assisted PRK and prophylactic corneal CXL in these patients seems to be a safe and effective option for managing visual rehabilitation [92].

A longer follow-up and larger case series are necessary to evaluate the safety, stability and efficacy of these procedures.

Conclusion

CXL using UVA light and using riboflavin as a photosensitizer creates new covalent crosslinks between collagen fibers. It has been demonstrated that CXL halts the progression of keratectasia in progressive keratoconus and post-LASIK corneas and tends to improve visual status. However, the complications make it necessary to improve the conventional procedure.

Attempts have been made to optimize CXL in order to minimize the potential for risk to corneas and to reduce patient discomfort. In fact, many lines of research are still under investigation to define the future of transepithelial CXL.

References

1 Andreassen TT, Simonsen AH, Oxlund H: Biomechanical properties of keratoconus and normal corneas. Exp Eye Res 1980;31:435–441.

2 Fawzy AS, Nitisusanta LI, Iqbal K, Daood U, Neo J: Riboflavin as a dentin crosslinking agent: ultraviolet A versus blue light. Dent Mater 2012;28:1284–1291.

3 Malik NS, Moss SJ, Ahmed N, Furth AJ, Wall RS, Meek KM: Ageing of the human corneal stroma: structural and biochemical changes. Biochim Biophys Acta 1992;1138:222–228.

4 Bailey AJ, Paul RG, Knott L: Mechanisms of maturation and ageing of collagen. Mech Ageing Dev 1998;106:1–56.

5 Sady C, Khosrof S, Nagaraj R: Advanced Maillard reaction and crosslinking of corneal collagen in diabetes. Biochem Biophys Res Commun 1995;214:793–797.

6 Wollensak G, Spoerl E, Seiler T: Riboflavin/ultraviolet-a-induced collagen crosslinking for the treatment of keratoconus. Am J Ophthalmol 2003;135:620–627.

7 Wollensak G: Crosslinking treatment of progressive keratoconus: new hope. Curr Opin Ophthalmol 2006;17:356–360.

8 Daxer A, Misof K, Grabner B, Ettl A, Fratzl P: Collagen fibrils in the human corneal stroma: structure and aging. Invest Ophthalmol Vis Sci 1998;39:644–648.

9 Kagan HM, Trackman PC: Properties and function of lysyl oxidase. Am J Respir Cell Mol Biol 1991;5:206–210.

10   Bykhovskaya Y, Li X, Epifantseva I, Haritunians T, Siscovick D, Aldave A, Szczotka-Flynn L, Iyengar SK, Taylor KD, Rotter JI, Rabinowitz YS: Variation in the lysyl oxidase (LOX) gene is associated with keratoconus in family-based and case-control studies. Invest Ophthalmol Vis Sci 2012;53:4152–4157.

11   Avetisov SE, Mamikonian VR, Novikov IA: [The role of tear acidity and Cu-cofactor of lysyl oxidase activity in the pathogenesis of keratoconus]. Vestn Oftalmol 2011;127:3–8.

12   Duan X, McLaughlin C, Griffith M, Sheardown H: Biofunctionalization of collagen for improved biological response: scaffolds for corneal tissue engineering. Biomaterials 2007;28:78–88.

13   Hurmeric V, Sahin A, Ozge G, Bayer A: The relationship between corneal biomechanical properties and confocal microscopy findings in normal and keratoconic eyes. Cornea 2010;29:641–649.

14   Liu R, Chu RY, Zhou XT, Qu XM, Dai JH, Wang L: [A compare study on cornea biomechanical properties in normal and keratoconic eyes]. Zhonghua Yan Ke Za Zhi 2009;45:509–513.

15   Terai N, Raiskup F, Haustein M, Pillunat LE, Spoerl E: Identification of biomechanical properties of the cornea: the ocular response analyzer. Curr Eye Res 2012;37:553–562.

16   Winkler M, Chai D, Kriling S, Nien CJ, Brown DJ, Jester B, Juhasz T, Jester JV: Nonlinear optical macroscopic assessment of 3-D corneal collagen organization and axial biomechanics. Invest Ophthalmol Vis Sci 2011;52:8818–8827.

17   Komai Y, Ushiki T: The three-dimensional organization of collagen fibrils in the human cornea and sclera. Invest Ophthalmol Vis Sci 1991;32:2244–2258.

18   Meek KM, Boote C: The organization of collagen in the corneal stroma. Exp Eye Res 2004;78:503–512.

19   Abahussin M, Hayes S, Knox Cartwright NE, Kamma-Lorger CS, Khan Y, Marshall J, Meek KM: 3D collagen orientation study of the human cornea using X-ray diffraction and femtosecond laser technology. Invest Ophthalmol Vis Sci 2009;50:5159–5164.

20   Saad A, Lteif Y, Azan E, Gatinel D: Biomechanical properties of keratoconus suspect eyes. Invest Ophthalmol Vis Sci 2010;51:2912–2916.

21   Tomkins O, Garzozi HJ: Collagen crosslinking: Strengthening the unstable cornea. Clin Ophthalmol 2008;2:863–867.

22   Spoerl E, Huhle M, Seiler T: Induction of cross-links in corneal tissue. Exp Eye Res 1998;66:97–103.

23   Zhang Y, Conrad AH, Conrad GW: Effects of ultraviolet-A and riboflavin on the interaction of collagen and proteoglycans during corneal cross-linking. J Biol Chem 2011;286:13011–13022.

24   Kamaev P, Friedman MD, Sherr E, Muller D: Photochemical kinetics of corneal cross-linking with riboflavin. Invest Ophthalmol Vis Sci 2012;53: 2360–2367.

25   Kopsachilis N, Tsaousis KT, Tsinopoulos IT, Kruse FE, Welge-Luessen U: A novel mechanism of UV-A and riboflavin-mediated corneal cross-linking through induction of tissue transglutaminases. Cornea 2013;32:1034–1039.

26   Raiskup-Wolf F, Hoyer A, Spoerl E, Pillunat LE: Collagen crosslinking with riboflavin and ultraviolet-A light in keratoconus: long-term results. J Cataract Refract Surg 2008;34:796–801.

27   Schumacher S, Mrochen M, Wernli J, Bueeler M, Seiler T: Optimization model for UV-riboflavin corneal cross-linking. Invest Ophthalmol Vis Sci 2012;53:762–769.

28   Spoerl E, Mrochen M, Sliney D, Trokel S, Seiler T: Safety of UVA-riboflavin cross-linking of the cornea. Cornea 2007;26:385–389.

29   Wollensak G, Iomdina E: Long-term biomechanical properties of rabbit cornea after photodynamic collagen crosslinking. Acta Ophthalmol 2009;87:48–51.

30   Spoerl E, Wollensak G, Seiler T: Increased resistance of crosslinked cornea against enzymatic digestion. Curr Eye Res 2004;29:35–40.

31   Wittig-Silva C, Whiting M, Lamoureux E, Lindsay RG, Sullivan LJ, Snibson GR: A randomized controlled trial of corneal collagen cross-linking in progressive keratoconus: preliminary results. J Refract Surg 2008;24:S720–S725.

32   Vinciguerra P, Albè E, Trazza S, Rosetta P, Vinciguerra R, Seiler T, Epstein D: Refractive, topographic, tomographic, and aberrometric analysis of keratoconic eyes undergoing corneal cross-linking. Ophthalmology 2009;116:369–378.

33   Caporossi A, Mazzotta C, Baiocchi S, Caporossi T: Long-term results of riboflavin ultraviolet a corneal collagen cross-linking for keratoconus in Italy: the Siena eye cross study. Am J Ophthalmol 2010;149:585–593.

34   Greenstein SA, Fry KL, Hersh PS: Corneal topography indices after corneal collagen crosslinking for keratoconus and corneal ectasia: one-year results. J Cataract Refract Surg 2011;37:1282–1290.

35   Hersh PS, Greenstein SA, Fry KL: Corneal collagen crosslinking for keratoconus and corneal ectasia: One-year results. J Cataract Refract Surg 2011;37: 149–160.

36   Raiskup F, Spoerl E: Corneal crosslinking with riboflavin and ultraviolet A. Part II. Clinical indications and results. Ocul Surf 2013;11:93–108.

37   Asri D, Touboul D, Fournié P, Malet F, Garra C, Gallois A, Malecaze F, Colin J: Corneal collagen crosslinking in progressive keratoconus: multicenter results from the French National Reference Center for Keratoconus. J Cataract Refract Surg 2011;37:2137–2143.

38   Koller T, Mrochen M, Seiler T: Complication and failure rates after corneal crosslinking. J Cataract Refract Surg 2009;35:1358–1362.

39   Seiler TG, Schmidinger G, Fischinger I, Koller T, Seiler T: [Complications of corneal cross-linking]. Ophthalmologe 2013;110:639–644.

40   Ghanem VC, Ghanem RC, de Oliveira R: Postoperative pain after corneal collagen cross-linking. Cornea 2013;32:20–24.

41   Raiskup F, Hoyer A, Spoerl E: Permanent corneal haze after riboflavin-UVA-induced cross-linking in keratoconus. J Refract Surg 2009;25:S824–S828.

42   Herrmann CI, Hammer T, Duncker GI: [Hazeformation (corneal scarring) after cross-linking therapy in keratoconus]. Ophthalmologe 2008;105:485–487.

43   Angunawela RI, Arnalich-Montiel F, Allan BD: Peripheral sterile corneal infiltrates and melting after collagen crosslinking for keratoconus. J Cataract Refract Surg 2009;35:606–607.

44   Pollhammer M, Cursiefen C: Bacterial keratitis early after corneal crosslinking with riboflavin and ultraviolet-A. J Cataract Refract Surg 2009;35:588–589.

45   Zamora KV, Males JJ: Polymicrobial keratitis after a collagen cross-linking procedure with postoperative use of a contact lens: a case report. Cornea 2009; 28:474–476.

46 Kymionis GD, Portaliou DM, Bouzoukis DI, Suh LH, Pallikaris AI, Markomanolakis M, Yoo SH: Herpetic keratitis with iritis after corneal crosslinking with riboflavin and ultraviolet A for keratoconus. J Cataract Refract Surg 2007;33:1982–1984.

47 Stanca HT, Tabacaru B: [The use of iontophoresis in corneal crosslinking technique]. Oftalmologia 2013;57:3–8.

48 Tao X, Yu H, Zhang Y, Li Z, Jhanji V, Ni S, Wang Y, Mu G: Role of corneal epithelium in riboflavin/ultraviolet-A mediated corneal cross-linking treatment in rabbit eyes. Biomed Res Int 2013; 2013:624563.

49 Baiocchi S, Mazzotta C, Cerretani D, Caporossi T, Caporossi A: Corneal crosslinking: riboflavin concentration in corneal stroma exposed with and without epithelium. J Cataract Refract Surg 2009;35:893–899.

50 Kissner A, Spoerl E, Jung R, Spekl K, Pillunat LE, Raiskup F: Pharmacological modification of the epithelial permeability by benzalkonium chloride in UVA/Riboflavin corneal collagen cross-linking. Curr Eye Res 2010;35:715–721.

51 Chang SW, Chi RF, Wu CC, Su MJ: Benzalkonium chloride and gentamicin cause a leak in corneal epithelial cell membrane. Exp Eye Res 2000;71:3–10.

52 Uematsu M, Kumagami T, Kusano M, Yamada K, Mishima K, Fujimura K, Sasaki H, Kitaoka T: Acute corneal epithelial change after instillation of benzalkonium chloride evaluated using a newly developed in vivo corneal transepithelial electric resistance measurement method. Ophthalmic Res 2007;39: 308–314.

53 Filippello M, Stagni E, O'Brart D: Transepithelial corneal collagen crosslinking: bilateral study. J Cataract Refract Surg 2012;38:283–291.

54 Caporossi A, Mazzotta C, Paradiso AL, Baiocchi S, Marigliani D, Caporossi T: Transepithelial corneal collagen crosslinking for progressive keratoconus: 24-month clinical results. J Cataract Refract Surg 2013;39:1157–1163.

55 Raiskup F, Pinelli R, Spoerl E: Riboflavin osmolar modification for transepithelial corneal cross-linking. Curr Eye Res 2012;37:234–238.

56 Martin J, Malreddy P, Iwamoto T, Freeman LC, Davidson HJ, Tomich JM, Schultz BD: NC-1059: a channel-forming peptide that modulates drug delivery across in vitro corneal epithelium. Invest Ophthalmol Vis Sci 2009;50:3337–3345.

57 Tyle P: Iontophoretic devices for drug delivery. Pharm Res 1986;3:318–326.

58 Selinger E: Iontophoresis with contract lens type and eyecup electrodes some points of the theory and technic of ion transfer. Arch Ophthal 1947;38:645–653.

59 Yoo SH, Dursun D, Dubovy S, Miller D, Alfonso E, Forster RK, Behar-Cohen F, Parel JM: Iontophoresis for the treatment of paecilomyces keratitis. Cornea 2002;21:131–132.

60 Costello CT, Jeske AH: Iontophoresis: applications in transdermal medication delivery. Phys Ther 1995;75:554–563.

61 Cassagne M, Laurent C, Rodrigues M, Galinier A, Spoerl E, Galiacy SD, Soler V, Fournié P, Malecaze F: Iontophoresis transcorneal delivery technique for transepithelial corneal collagen crosslinking with riboflavin in a rabbit model. Invest Ophthalmol Vis Sci DOI: 10.1167/iovs.13-12595.

62 Daxer A, Mahmoud HA, Venkateswaran RS: Corneal crosslinking and visual rehabilitation in keratoconus in one session without epithelial debridement: new technique. Cornea 2010;29:1176–1179. doi: 10.1097/ICO.0b013e3181d2c644.

63 Dong Z, Zhou X: Collagen cross-linking with riboflavin in a femtosecond laser-created pocket in rabbit corneas: 6-month results. Am J Ophthalmol 2011;152:22–27.e1.

64 Zhang ZY, Hoffman MR: Collagen cross-linking with riboflavin in a femtosecond laser-created pocket in rabbit corneas. Am J Ophthalmol 2011;152: 1082–1083; author reply 1083–1084.

65 Kanellopoulos AJ: Collagen cross-linking in early keratoconus with riboflavin in a femtosecond laser-created pocket: initial clinical results. J Refract Surg 2009;25:1034–1037.

66 Wernli J, Schumacher S, Spoerl E, Mrochen M: The efficacy of corneal cross-linking shows a sudden decrease with very high intensity UV light and short treatment time. Invest Ophthalmol Vis Sci 2013;54:1176–1180.

67 Schumacher S, Oeftiger L, Mrochen M: Equivalence of biomechanical changes induced by rapid and standard corneal cross-linking, using riboflavin and ultraviolet radiation. Invest Ophthalmol Vis Sci 2011;52:9048–9052.

68 Beshtawi IM, O'Donnell C, Radhakrishnan H: Biomechanical properties of corneal tissue after ultraviolet-A-riboflavin crosslinking. J Cataract Refract Surg 2013;39:451–462.

69 Touboul D, Efron N, Smadja D, Praud D, Malet F, Colin J: Corneal confocal microscopy following conventional, transepithelial, and accelerated corneal collagen cross-linking procedures for keratoconus. J Refract Surg 2012;28: 769–776.

70 Cınar Y, Cingü AK, Turkcu FM, Yüksel H, Sahin A, Yıldırım A, Caca I, Cınar T: Accelerated corneal collagen cross-linking for progressive keratoconus. Cutan Ocul Toxicol 2014;33:168–171.

71 Friedman MD, Pertaub R, Usher D, Sherr E, Kamaev P, Muller D: Advanced corneal cross-linking system with fluorescence dosimetry. J Ophthalmol 2012; 2012:303459.

72 Spoerl E, Wollensak G, Reber F, Pillunat L: Cross-linking of human amniotic membrane by glutaraldehyde. Ophthalmic Res 2004;36:71–77.

73 Avila MY, Gerena VA, Navia JL: Corneal crosslinking with genipin, comparison with UV-riboflavin in ex-vivo model. Mol Vis 2012;18:1068–1073.

74 Avila MY, Navia JL: Effect of genipin collagen crosslinking on porcine corneas. J Cataract Refract Surg 2010;36: 659–664.

75 Cherfan D, Verter EE, Melki S, Gisel TE, Doyle FJ Jr, Scarcelli G, Yun SH, Redmond RW, Kochevar IE: Collagen crosslinking using rose bengal and green light to increase corneal stiffness. Invest Ophthalmol Vis Sci 2013;54:3426–3433.

76 Rabinowitz YS: Keratoconus. Surv Ophthalmol 1998;42:297–319.

77 Li G, Fan ZJ, Peng XJ: Corneal collagen crosslinking for corneal ectasia of post-LASIK: one-year results. Int J Ophthalmol 2012;5:190–195.

78 Yam JC, Cheng AC: Prognostic factors for visual outcomes after crosslinking for keratoconus and post-LASIK ectasia. Eur J Ophthalmol 2013;23:799–806.

79 Ghanem RC, Santhiago MR, Berti TB, Thomaz S, Netto MV: Collagen cross-linking with riboflavin and ultraviolet-A in eyes with pseudophakic bullous keratopathy. J Cataract Refract Surg 2010;36:273–276.

80 Sharma N, Roy S, Maharana PK, Sehra SV, Sinha R, Tandon R, Titiyal JS, Vajpayee RB: Outcomes of corneal collagen crosslinking in pseudophakic bullous keratopathy. Cornea 2014;33:243–246.

81 Skaat A, Zadok D, Goldich Y, Varssano D, Berger Y, Ezra-Nimni O, Avni I, Barequet IS: Riboflavin/UVA photochemical therapy for severe infectious keratitis. Eur J Ophthalmol 2014;24:21–28.

82 Hayes S, Kamma-Lorger CS, Boote C, Young RD, Quantock AJ, Rost A, Khatib Y, Harris J, Yagi N, Terrill N, Meek KM: The effect of riboflavin/UVA collagen cross-linking therapy on the structure and hydrodynamic behaviour of the ungulate and rabbit corneal stroma. PLoS One 2013;8:e52860.

83 Arance-Gil Á, Gutiérrez-Ortega ÁR, Villa-Collar C, Nieto-Bona A, Lopes-Ferreira D, González-Méijome JM: Corneal cross-linking for Acanthamoeba keratitis in an orthokeratology patient after swimming in contaminated water. Cont Lens Anterior Eye 2014;37:224–227.

84 Kymionis GD, Kontadakis GA, Kounis GA, Portaliou DM, Karavitaki AE, Magarakis M, Yoo S, Pallikaris IG: Simultaneous topography-guided PRK followed by corneal collagen cross-linking for keratoconus. J Refract Surg 2009;25:S807–S811.

85 Al-Tuwairqi W, Sinjab MM: Intracorneal ring segments implantation followed by same-day topography-guided PRK and corneal collagen CXL in low to moderate keratoconus. J Refract Surg 2013;29:59–63.

86 Kılıç A, Kamburoglu G, Akıncı A: Riboflavin injection into the corneal channel for combined collagen crosslinking and intrastromal corneal ring segment implantation. J Cataract Refract Surg 2012;38:878–883.

87 Legare ME, Iovieno A, Yeung SN, Lichtinger A, Kim P, Hollands S, Slomovic AR, Rootman DS: Intacs with or without same-day corneal collagen cross-linking to treat corneal ectasia. Can J Ophthalmol 2013;48:173–178.

88 Yeung SN, Ku JY, Lichtinger A, Low SA, Kim P, Rootman DS: Efficacy of single or paired intrastromal corneal ring segment implantation combined with collagen crosslinking in keratoconus. J Cataract Refract Surg 2013;39:1146–1151.

89 Kremer I, Aizenman I, Lichter H, Shayer S, Levinger S: Simultaneous wavefront-guided photorefractive keratectomy and corneal collagen crosslinking after intrastromal corneal ring segment implantation for keratoconus. J Cataract Refract Surg 2012;38:1802–1807.

90 Yeung SN, Low SA, Ku JY, Lichtinger A, Kim P, Teichman J, Iovieno A, Rootman DS: Transepithelial phototherapeutic keratectomy combined with implantation of a single inferior intrastromal corneal ring segment and collagen crosslinking in keratoconus. J Cataract Refract Surg 2013;39:1152–1156.

91 Lin DT, Holland S, Tan JC, Moloney G: Clinical results of topography-based customized ablations in highly aberrated eyes and keratoconus/ectasia with cross-linking. J Refract Surg 2012;28(11 Suppl):S841–S848.

92 Spadea L, Paroli M: Simultaneous topography-guided PRK followed by corneal collagen cross-linking after lamellar keratoplasty for keratoconus. Clin Ophthalmol 2012;6:1793–1800.

Prof. François Malecaze
Department of Ophthalmology, Purpan Hospital
1 place du Dr Baylac
FR–31059 Toulouse (France)
E-Mail malecaze.fr@chu-toulouse.fr

Güell JL (ed): Cornea. ESASO Course Series. Basel, Karger, 2015, vol 6, pp 66–73
DOI: 10.1159/000381493

Actual Indications for Intracorneal Ring Segment Implantation in Keratoconus

George D. Kymionis

Vardinoyiannion Eye Institute of Crete (VEIC), Faculty of Medicine, University of Crete, Heraklion, Crete, Greece; Bascom Palmer Eye Institute, Miller School of Medicine, University of Miami, Miami, Fla., USA

Abstract

Intracorneal ring segments (ICRS) are small synthetic implements designed to achieve refractive adjustment by flattening the cornea. Three common types of commercially available ICRS are Intacs, Keraring and Ferrara rings. Low myopia was the initial indication for implantation of ICRS, and indications later included ectatic corneal diseases (such as keratoconus and pellucid marginal degeneration) and ectasia after laser-assisted in situ keratomileusis. Two surgical procedures are used for implantation of ICRS: a mechanical technique, performed using two manual semicircular dissectors, and a femtosecond laser technique, performed with the assistance of femtosecond laser photodisruption for tunnel creation. The design parameters of ICRS, such as shape, thickness and diameter, have different effects on corneal curvature. Several nomograms have been developed in order to improve the outcome of refractive correction, depending on centration of the cone, corneal steepness and refraction. Implantation of ICRS is minimally invasive, although intraoperative and postoperative complications have been reported, depending on the surgical procedure. Combination with other treatment modalities, such as corneal collagen crosslinking and/or photorefractive keratectomy, has also been reported.

Introduction

Keratoconus is a progressive, noninflammatory ectatic disorder of the cornea that results in significant protrusion and thinning that are typically diagnosed during the second decade of life. The main symptoms are increasing irregular astigmatism and a decrease in best-corrected visual acuity. Corneal topography may reveal the disease early and is very useful in detecting progression. Inferior corneal steepening is the most common topographic finding. Management of keratoconus includes the use of glasses and contact lenses for visual rehabilitation at early stages, corneal collagen crosslinking (CXL) in the case of progression to achieve stabilization and penetrating or deep lamellar keratoplasty in advanced cases.

Intracorneal ring segments (ICRS) are implanted deep into the corneal stroma and were originally used to treat low to moderate myopia [1, 2]. Currently, they are used to manage ectatic corneal disorders such as keratoconus [3, 4], pellucid marginal degeneration [5] and ectasia after laser-assisted in situ keratomileusis (LASIK) [6].

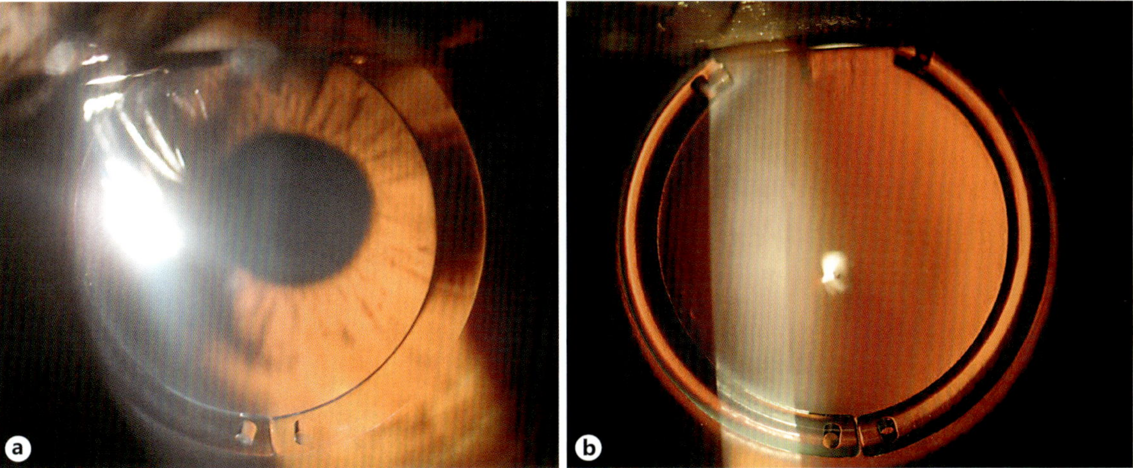

Fig. 1. Slit-lamp photo of a patient implanted with intracorneal rings (Intacs) (**a**) with wide illumination and (**b**) with retroillumination.

Intracorneal Ring Segments: Types and Materials

Intrastromal corneal ring segments are polymethyl methacrylate implants that are implanted at the midperipheral corneal stroma in order to flatten the central corneal zone. There are three types of ICRS commercially available: Intacs (Addition Technologies Inc., Fremont, California, USA), Keraring (Mediphacos, Belo Horizonte, Brazil) and Ferrara rings (Ferrara Ophthalmics, Belo Horizonte, Brazil). Ferrara rings have a smaller optical zone and more of a flattening effect than Intacs does.

Indications for Intracorneal Ring Segment Implantation in Keratoconus

Implantation of intracorneal rings is indicated in ectatic corneas when visual acuity cannot be improved with spectacle correction. Patients with keratoconus, post-LASIK ectasia or pellucid marginal degeneration may be treated. In these patients, contact lens intolerance is also an indication since implantation of intracorneal rings has been shown to improve visual acuity and tolerance of contact lens wear.

In order to be successful, intracorneal ring implantation should be implemented in corneas with a clear optical zone and a corneal thickness >450 μm in the area of implantation. Intrastromal corneal ring segments are inserted in intrastromal channels (created either manually or with femtosecond (FS) lasers) at a depth of 75% of the thinnest pachymetry (fig. 1).

Surgical Techniques for Intracorneal Ring Segment Implantation

Mechanical Technique

Topical anesthesia is performed, and the center of the cornea is located. A marker is used to mark the sites and the incision points on the steep axis of the cornea. A diamond knife is set to a depth between 70 and 80% of the corneal thickness measured by ultrasound corneal pachymetry. A radial incision of 1.2–1.8 mm width is created in the marked position. Pocketing hooks create corneal pockets on each side at the bottom of the incision. A vacuum system is started after a suction ring is placed around the limbus. Two semicircular dissectors are placed (one clockwise and the other counter-clockwise) into the pocket and are advanced by rotational movement, creating two semicircular tunnels with specific diameters. Ring segments may be placed into the tunnels at least 1 mm away from the incision.

Femtosecond Laser Technique
The surgical procedure with an FS laser is also performed under topical anesthesia. The disposable suction ring of the FS laser system is centered after marking a reference point on the cornea (pupil center or first Purkinje reflex) and measuring the corneal thickness at the area of implantation (5- or 6-mm diameter). The disposable glass lens is applanated to the cornea to fixate the eye and to help to maintain the precise distance from the laser head to the focal point. An entry cut with the FS laser is created in order to allow access ring placement in the tunnel. Ring segments are inserted into the created tunnels (pupil center or first Purkinje reflex) at approximately 70–80% of the corneal thickness.

Compared to the manual technique, the FS laser makes tunnel creation easy, quick and more reproducible and also offers accurate tunnel dimensions (width, diameter and depth) [7]. With mechanical dissectors, the segment depth may be shallower at positions further from the incision. Theoretically, compared with mechanical tunnel creation, which relies on the surgeon's skills, the FS laser-assisted procedure should generate more accurate stromal dissection, leading to better visual and refractive results.

However, similar visual and refractive outcomes were reported for the two procedures in a short-term follow-up of eyes effected by keratoconus or post-LASIK ectasia [8, 9].

Kubaloglu et al. [10] compared the clinical outcomes of keratoconic patients treated with Keraring to those of patients treated with Intacs. Both implants were safe and effective. No difference was recorded in visual or refractive outcomes when comparing mechanically and FS la-

ser-created channels. However, it was reported that use of the FS laser made the procedure faster, easier and more comfortable. Further experience and the development of more accurate nomograms should improve clinical outcomes.

Mechanism of Action

The implantation of ICRS results in redistribution of the corneal peripheral lamellae, producing flattening of the central cornea and decreasing refractive disorders, myopia and astigmatism [4]. The effect is proportional to the implant's thickness and inversely proportional to the implant's diameter [2]. The refractive result of the surgical intervention is possibly reversible since the ring segments can be explanted and replaced with ring segments of a different thickness to produce a different result. Unlike with surface ablation or LASIK, the central clear zone of the cornea is not directly treated. The normal cornea is generally prolate, or steeper centrally than peripherally. The ring segments flatten the peripheral cornea more than the central cornea, and therefore, the central cornea profile is maintained after placement of the ring segments. This is important because it has been suggested that a prolate cornea may minimize glare and halo symptoms. Additionally, since the ring segments are narrow, the overlying stroma can receive nutrients from surrounding tissue (fig. 2–4).

Nomogram for Intracorneal Ring Segment Implantation

Currently, several different nomograms have been published in the literature regarding the best choice of ICRS in each case. Authors have used either one or preferably two symmetrical or asymmetrical rings implanted in the horizontal, vertical or oblique position in order to achieve the best possible correction. There are also nomograms proposed by the manufacturers of

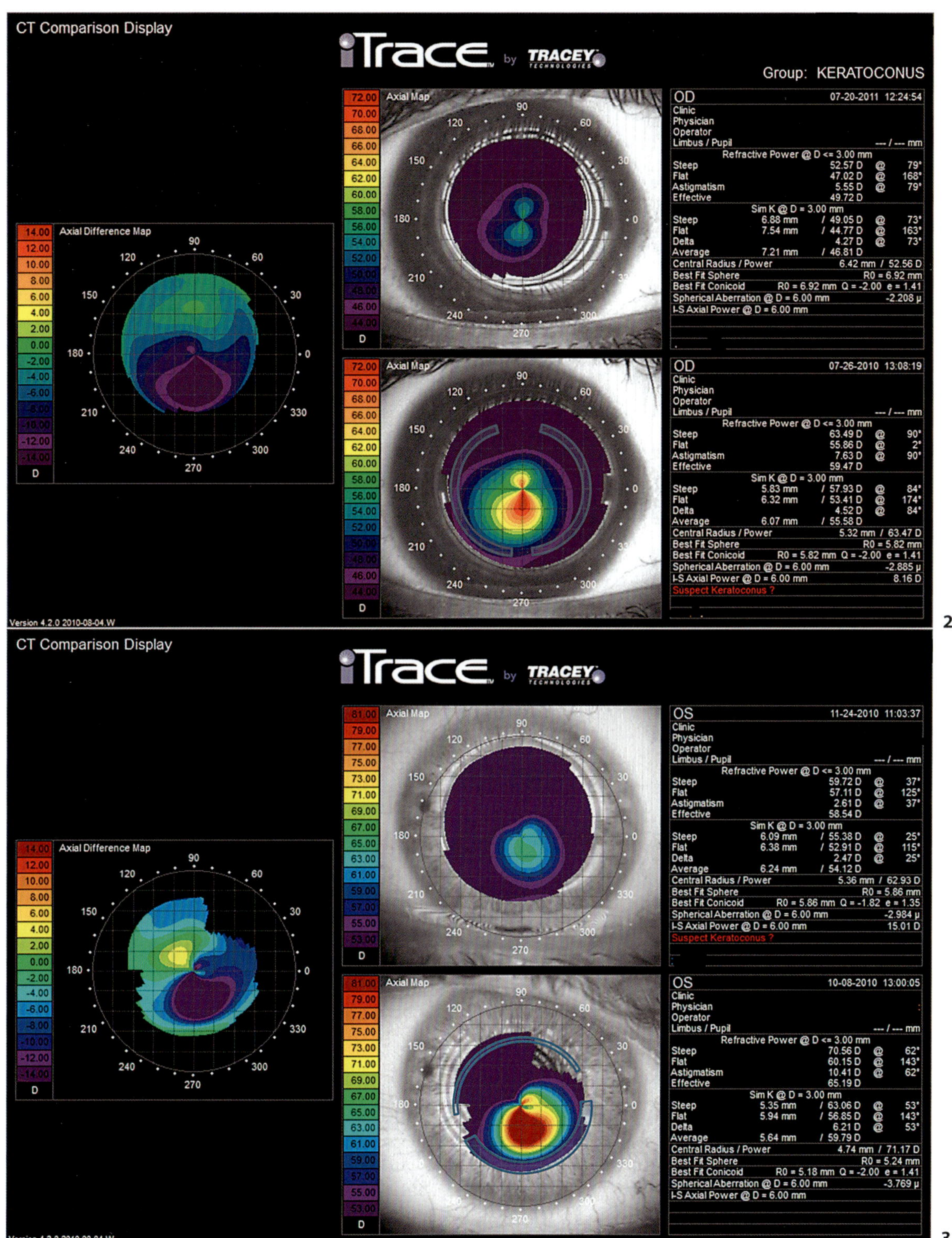

(For legend see next page.)

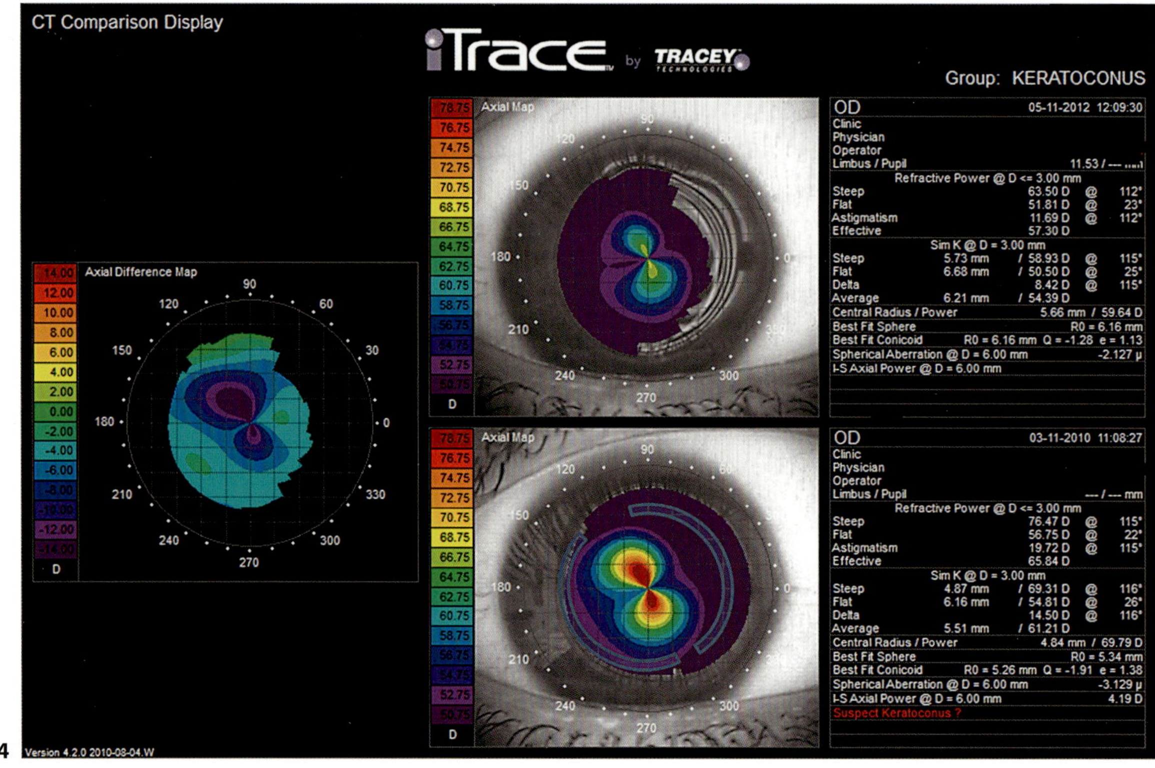

Fig. 2–4. Axial topography maps of patients who were treated with Intacs implantation. Prior to treatment (bottom right), after treatment (top right) and difference map (left). On the prior-to-treatment map (bottom right) of each image, there is a schematic representation of the ring position.

ICRS. The choice of implant in each case depends on the shape and position of the cone and on the refraction. For Intacs, it is proposed that two rings of the same size should be implanted in the central cone and that two rings with different sizes should be implanted when the cone is located outside the 3.5-mm central zone or when astigmatism is greater than a cylinder. The size of both rings in the case of symmetrical implantation and the size of the inferior ring in the case of asymmetrical implantation depend on the amount of desired refractive correction. Ferrara rings are available in different arc lengths, diameters and segment thicknesses. All of these parameters are adjusted for each case according to the shape and condition of the cone and according to corneal asphericity.

Example Cases

Case 1

The patient presented with manifest refraction of –3.00–6.25X175°. His keratometry was K1: 57.93@84° and K2: 53.41@174°. According to corneal topography, he had a central cone with relatively symmetrical astigmatism. He was implanted with two Intacs SK rings of 0.350-mm thickness, which were placed nasotemporally through a superior incision on the steep meridian. His manifest refraction 6 months post-treatment was +1.00–3.75X160 (fig. 2).

Case 2

The patient presented with manifest refraction of –4.25–7.50X130°. His keratometry was K1:

Kymionis

63.06@53° and K2: 56.85@143°. According to corneal topography, he had an inferior asymmetric cone. He was implanted with two Intacs rings with different thicknesses, which were placed superoinferiorly (embracing the steep axis) through an incision on the steep meridian. The inferior ring had a thickness of 0.450 mm, and the superior ring had a thickness of 0.210 mm. His manifest refraction 6 months post-treatment was −3.25–1.75X10° (fig. 3).

Case 3

The patient presented with manifest refraction of −9.25–10.00X20°. His keratometry was K1: 69.31@116° and K2: 54.81@26°. According to corneal topography, he had a central cone with relatively symmetrical astigmatism on the oblique axis. He was implanted with two Intacs SK rings of 0.450-mm thickness, which were placed obliquely nasotemporally (embracing the steep axis) through a superior incision on the steep meridian. His manifest refraction 6 months post-treatment was −3.25–6.25X25° (fig. 4).

Complications of Intracorneal Ring Segment Implantation

Complications associated with the mechanical technique consist of epithelial defects, anterior or posterior perforation by the mechanical spreader, shallow or uneven placement of the ICRS, decentration, extension of the incision toward the central cornea or limbus and corneal stromal edema around the incision and channel due to surgical manipulation [11, 12]. Most cases of extrusion have been observed in eyes that underwent implantation using mechanical dissection, although three cases of ring extrusion in advanced keratoconus and one case of segment migration to the incision site have been reported using the FS laser-assisted procedure for channel creation [12].

Coskunseven et al. [13] reported complications after the implantation of intrastromal ring segments in keratoconic patients using the IntraLase FS laser, stating that incomplete channel creation (intraoperatively) and segment migration (postoperatively) were the most common complications. The study demonstrated that galvanometer lag error (0.6%), endothelial perforation (0.6%) and vacuum loss (0.1%) were additional intraoperative adverse events and that superficial movement of the segments (0.1%), corneal melting (0.2%) and infection (0.1%) were postoperative complications. Moreover, corneal vascularization in patients implanted with Intacs, either with or without concomitant contact lens wear, has been reported [14, 15] (fig. 5).

Combination of Intracorneal Rings with Other Surgical Procedures

Lately, the combination of CXL with photorefractive keratectomy (PRK) has been shown to be an effective solution for the visual rehabilitation of patients with keratoconus [16–18]. In order to improve the efficacy of these methods even more and to expand their applications, they have been combined with the implantation of ICRS in several studies. In most of the studies, the first step of the procedure is the implantation of the ICRS, and after a sufficient interval in order for the refraction to stabilize, PRK and CXL are applied, either in combination or sequentially (fig. 6).

Fig. 5. a Slit-lamp photo of a patient 10 years after Intacs implantation. The patient presented with severe central corneal neovascularization 5 years after starting contact lens use. **b** Slit-lamp photo of the patient's eye 1 month after discontinuing contact lens use, showing recession of the neovascularization.
Fig. 6. Axial topography maps of a patient who was treated with Intacs implantation and who underwent simultaneous topo-guided photorefractive keratectomy and corneal collagen crosslinking after 1 year. Prior to Intacs implantation (top right), after Intacs implantation (middle left) and after simultaneous topo-guided photorefractive keratectomy and corneal collagen crosslinking (bottom right) and corresponding difference maps (left).

(For figure see next page.)

5
a
b

6
iTrace by TRACEY TECHNOLOGIES
Axial Difference Map
Axial Difference Map
3.72 mm
197°
Axial Map
OD
03-15-2010 12:29:06
Clinic
Physician
Operator
Limbus / Pupil --- / --- mm
Refractive Power @ D <= 3.00 mm
Steep
Flat
Astigmatism
Effective
Sim K @ D = 3.00 mm
Steep 5.61 mm / 60.18 D @ 111°
Flat 6.23 mm / 54.14 D @ 21°
Delta 6.04 D @ 111°
Average 5.92 mm / 57.00 D
Central Radius / Power 5.12 mm / 65.93 D
Best Fit Sphere R0 = 5.62 mm
Best Fit Conicoid R0 = 5.62 mm Q = -0.40 e = 0.63
Spherical Aberration @ D = 6.00 mm -1.099 µ
I-S Axial Power @ D = 6.00 mm
OD
08-26-2010 13:20:35
Clinic
Physician
Operator
Limbus / Pupil --- / --- mm
Refractive Power @ D <= 3.00 mm
Steep
Flat
Astigmatism
Effective
Sim K @ D = 3.00 mm
Steep 6.37 mm / 52.95 D @ 93°
Flat 6.96 mm / 48.46 D @ 3°
Delta 4.48 D @ 93°
Average 6.67 mm / 50.61 D
Central Radius / Power 5.65 mm / 59.68 D
Best Fit Sphere R0 = 6.15 mm
Best Fit Conicoid R0 = 6.15 mm Q = -2.00 e = 1.41
Spherical Aberration @ D = 6.00 mm -3.311 µ
I-S Axial Power @ D = 6.00 mm
OD
03-27-2012 10:00:17
Clinic
Physician
Operator
Limbus / Pupil 12.13 / --- mm
Refractive Power @ D <= 3.00 mm
Steep
Flat
Astigmatism
Effective
Sim K @ D = 3.00 mm
Steep 6.69 mm / 50.48 D @ 143°
Flat 6.89 mm / 49.00 D @ 53°
Delta 1.47 D @ 143°
Average 6.79 mm / 49.73 D
Central Radius / Power 6.57 mm / 51.37 D
Best Fit Sphere R0 = 7.07 mm
Best Fit Conicoid R0 = 6.49 mm Q = -1.71 e = 1.31
Spherical Aberration @ D = 6.00 mm -0.818 µ
I-S Axial Power @ D = 6.00 mm

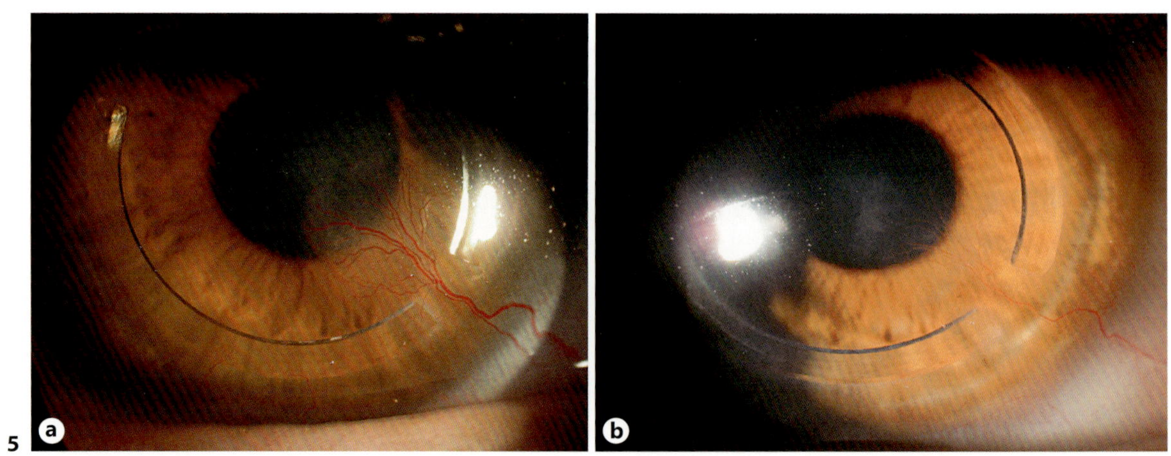

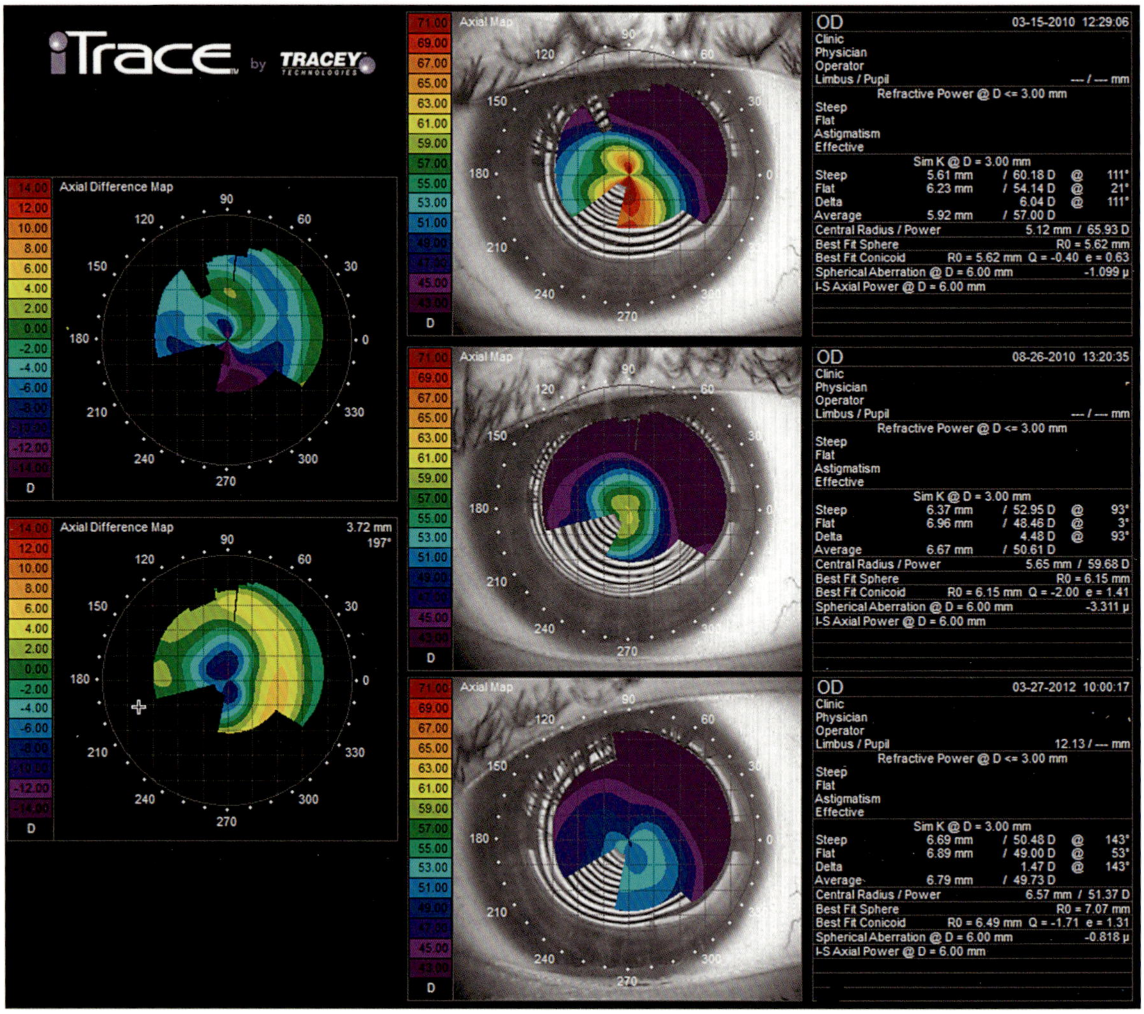

Conclusion

Intracorneal ring implantation may significantly improve the visual acuity and topography of patients with ectatic corneal disorders. The procedure of implantation performed with a FS laser has very few complications and is also reversible. In addition, it can be combined with PRK and CXL, thus offering patients the optimal refractive result that can be surgically achieved as well as postoperative stability.

References

1 Schanzlin DJ, Asbell PA, Burris TE, et al: The intrastromal corneal ring segments; phase II results for the correction of myopia. Ophthalmology 1997;104:1067–1078.
2 Patel S, Marshall J, Fitzke FWI: Model for deriving the optical performance of the myopic eye corrected with an intracorneal ring. J Refract Surg 1995;11:248–252.
3 Alio JL, Shabayek MH, Belda JI, et al: Analysis of results related to good and bad outcomes of Intacs implantation for keratoconus correction. J Cataract Refract Surg 2006;32:756–761.
4 Alio JL, Artola A, Ruiz-Moreno JM, et al: Changes in keratoconic corneas after intracorneal ring segment explantation and reimplantation. Ophthalmology 2004;111:747–751.
5 Pinero DP, Alio JL, Morbelli H, et al: Refractive and corneal aberrometric changes after intracorneal ring implantation in corneas with pellucid marginal degeneration. Ophthalmology 2009;116:1656–1664.
6 Pinero DP, Alio JL, Uceda-Montanes A, et al: Intracorneal ring segment implantation in corneas with postlaser in situ keratomileusis keratectasia. Ophthalmology 2009;116:1665–1674.
7 Lai MM, Tang M, Andrade EMM, et al: Optical coherence tomography to assess intrastromal ring segment depth in keratoconic eyes. J Cataract Refract Surg 2006;32:1860–1865.
8 Pinero D, Alio L: Intracorneal ring segments in ectatic corneal disease-a review. Clin Exp Ophthalmol 2010;38:154–167.
9 Rabinowitz YS, Li X, Ignacio TS, et al: Intacs inserts using the femtosecond laser compared to the mechanical spreader in the treatment of keratoconus. J Refract Surg 2006;22:764–771.
10 Kubaloglu A, Cinar Y, Sari ES, et al: Comparison of 2 intrastromal corneal ring segment models in the management of keratoconus. J Cataract Refract Surg 2010;36:978–985.
11 Kanellopoulos AJ, Pe LH, Perry HD, et al: Modified intracorneal ring segment implantations (Intacs) for the management of moderate to advanced keratoconus; efficiency and complications. Cornea 2006;25:29–33.
12 Boxer Wachler BS, Christie JP, Chandra NS, et al: Intacs for keratoconus. Ophthalmology 2003;110:1031–1040.
13 Coscunseven E, Kymionis GD, Tsiklis NS, et al: Complications of intrastromal corneal ring segment implantation using a femtosecond laser for channel creation: a survey of 850 eyes with keratoconus. Acta Ophthalmologica 2011;89:54–57.
14 Cosar CB, Sridhar MS, Sener B: Late onset of deep corneal vascularization: a rare complication of intrastromal corneal ring segments for keratoconus. Eur J Ophthalmol 2009;19:298–300.
15 Kymionis GD, Kontadakis GA: Severe corneal vascularization after intacs implantation and rigid contact lens use for the treatment of keratoconus. Semin Ophthalmol 2012;27:19–21.
16 Al-Tuwairqi W, Sinjab MM: Intracorneal ring segments implantation followed by same-day topography-guided PRK and corneal collagen CXL in low to moderate keratoconus. J Refract Surg 2013;29:59–63.
17 Coskunseven E, Jankov MR 2nd, Grentzelos MA, et al: Topography-guided transepithelial PRK after intracorneal ring segments implantation and corneal collagen CXL in a three-step procedure for keratoconus. J Refract Surg 2013;29:54–58.
18 Iovieno A, Légaré ME, Rootman DB, et al: Intracorneal ring segments implantation followed by same-day photorefractive keratectomy and corneal collagen cross-linking in keratoconus. J Refract Surg 2011;27:915–918.

George D. Kymionis, MD, PhD
Vardinoyiannion Eye Institute of Crete (VEIC)
University of Crete, Faculty of Medicine
GR–71003 Heraklion, Crete (Greece)
E-Mail kymionis@med.uoc.gr

Güell JL (ed): Cornea. ESASO Course Series. Basel, Karger, 2015, vol 6, pp 74–80
DOI: 10.1159/000381494

High-Risk Corneal Transplantation

Thomas A. Fuchsluger · Friedrich E. Kruse

University Hospital Erlangen, Friedrich-Alexander University Erlangen-Nuremberg, Department of Ophthalmology, Erlangen, Germany

Abstract

This chapter focuses on endeavors to perform keratoplasties to treat eyes in high-risk settings and discusses alternative approaches (such as lamellar strategies). The historical and molecular backgrounds (histocompatibility antigens) as well as associated risk factors (corneal neovascularization, ocular surface pathologies, re-keratoplasty, the size of a corneal graft, intraocular surgery, anterior segment inflammation, herpes simplex, patient age) are explained. Postoperative management includes treatment of herpes simplex, systemic treatment in high-risk settings and donor tissue selection with human leukocyte antigen matching. Lamellar keratoplasties are discussed as alternatives to conventional penetrating keratoplasties. The advantages and disadvantages of both anterior and posterior lamellar keratoplasties are highlighted.   © 2015 S. Karger AG, Basel

Introduction

Corneal transplantations are the most successful and frequently performed tissue transplantations in the world. The overall number of transplantations performed worldwide is estimated to be about 200,000 per year. In Europe, about 20–25,000 keratoplasties are performed each year [1], and about 55–60,000 are conducted in the United States [2].

The surgical outcome, however, strongly depends on the state of the patient's cornea prior to transplantation; low-risk settings can be distinguished from high-risk settings.

A *low-risk setting* is characterized by a nonvascularized patient cornea and the absence of corneal inflammation in the present or past. *High-risk settings*, in contrast, show vascularized corneal beds, e.g. as a result of corneal infection or inflammation of one or multiple corneal layers. In addition, pathological alteration of the anterior chamber, e.g. anterior synechia, glaucoma or chronic tear film instability, can be associated with a reduction in graft survival. By definition, every re-graft due to immunological graft failure is a high-risk keratoplasty. While low-risk keratoplasties show a success rate of over 90% after 2 years [3], the rates of rejection of high-risk keratoplasties can be up to 70% [4, 5]. Interestingly, such high rejection rates occur even under strong topical and systemic immunosuppression.

Historical Background

The first penetrating keratoplasty (pKP) was performed in 1906 by Eduard Zirm [6]. Interestingly, the first publications on graft rejection were published over 40 years later by Paufique [7] and Maumenee [8]. By that time, it had been observed that allografts of solid organs had a higher probability of failing compared to an allograft of a cornea. This observation led to the concept of the cornea being an immune-privileged site [8]. In the 1970s, Silverstein and Khodadoust detected antigens released by corneal grafts after transplantation and demonstrated that the host can respond to these antigens with an immune response. This process can result in corneal graft rejection [9, 10]. Corneal neovascularization of a patient's corneal bed results in compromised immune privilege and therefore leads to increased graft failure due to immune reaction.

Histocompatibility Antigens

As in solid organ transplantation, each graft expresses an individualized, characteristic pattern of molecules on the surface of the tissues (so-called 'transplantation antigens'). As some transplantation antigens produce a more intense immune response than others, these antigens have been sub-classified as 'major' and 'minor' [11]. Tissue randomly selected for transplantation will therefore result in the engraftment of a different pattern of (allogeneic) transplantation antigens. Therefore, the host organism will recognize the transplanted tissue as foreign and will initiate an immune response.

The 'major' transplantation antigens are termed 'human leukocyte antigens' (HLAs), and their genes are located in the 'major histocompatibility complex' (MHC). There are two 'classes' of 'major' transplantation antigens (HLAs): class I and class II. Class I antigens, which are transmembrane glycoproteins, are named HLA-A, HLA-B and HLA-C. These are expressed in different cell-specific quantities on most cells containing nuclei (such as corneal endothelial cells, keratocytes and epithelial cells) and on platelets. Class II antigens are found on certain immune

cells, such as antigen-presenting cells, Langerhans cells of the epithelium, macrophages and B cells. Typically, HLA-D genes determine the expression of these antigens (HLA-DP, HLA-DQ and HLA-DR) [12].

The 'minor' transplantation antigens derive from gene loci outside the MHC, and their genes are spread throughout the entire genome. Only when processed by MHC class I or class II molecules do these 'minor' transplantation antigens appear on the surface of allogeneic cells. An example of these 'minor' transplantation antigens is the ABO blood group antigens, which are also expressed by corneal epithelial cells.

Risk Factors for a High-Risk Transplantation Setting

Corneal Neovascularization
Vascularization of a host corneal bed is the predominant risk factor threatening the outcome of a transplanted cornea. Multiple authors have demonstrated that avascular corneal beds lead to significantly greater graft survival than vascularized corneal beds do [13, 14]. According to the 'Collaborative Corneal Transplantation Studies', two or more vascularized quadrants are defined as a 'high-risk setting' [15]. The rate of graft survival was reduced by about 50% when all four quadrants showed vascularization. Interestingly, vascularization also affected the probability of corneal endothelial rejection: about every third patient with a vascularized corneal bed displayed signs of endothelial immune rejection. However, only every seventh patient showed such endothelial rejection, with little or no neovascularization prior to keratoplasty [13]. Additionally, the depth of corneal neovessels is relevant: deep stromal neovascularization leads to a higher rate of graft rejection than superficial corneal neovascularization does [15, 16].

The degree of vascularization also affects the average duration until grafted corneas demonstrate signs of rejection. In extensively neovascularized corneal beds, the period without such a complication was merely 2 months. In mild neovascularization, the duration was 4 months, whereas vessel-free host corneas were without rejection symptoms for an average of 10 months following surgery [17].

The presence of pathological vessels in the corneal host bed also has an impact on the likelihood of successful treatment of a corneal rejection episode. Corneal transplants grafted in avascular corneal beds can be successfully treated in about two thirds of all cases, whereas only every second corneal rejection can be reversed in patients with preoperatively vascularized corneas [18].

Ocular Surface Pathologies
Diseases of the ocular surface endanger the integrity of a grafted donor cornea. Anomalies of the lids, the lacrimal gland or the glands supporting the tear film negatively impair tear film stability and the film's nutrition of the donor cornea [19]. Restoration of lid pathologies (e.g. entropion) and improvement of the tear film situation (e.g. insertion of punctual plugs into the superior and/or inferior lacrimal punctae and eventual cauterization of the lacrimal punctae) are of utmost importance prior to any surgery on the cornea.

More severe ocular surface diseases, including chemical injuries, often lead to limbal stem cell deficiency and endanger the integrity and survival of a corneal graft, as do systemic pathologies like Stevens-Johnson syndrome or cicatricial pemphigoid. Corneal transplantation in these very cases is either contraindicated or requires a specific approach. This approach can be restoration of the ocular surface, e.g. using keratolimbal allografts [20]. However, high rates of corneal rejection are reported, regardless of whether the keratolimbal allograft and the pKP are performed in one or two steps. An alternative approach is the performance of limbal keratoplasty [21]. Here, the survival rates are considerably higher than with conventional pKP, as vital donor limbus is transplanted onto the ocular surface following superficial lamellar keratectomy (up to 65% in a 5-year follow-up, depending on the number of mismatches in the graft).

Re-Keratoplasty
Once an earlier pKP fails due to immunological graft rejection, the prognosis of each subsequent full-thickness graft is considerably worse [14, 22]. Graft survival in vascularized corneal beds is about 60% following one episode of graft rejection, merely 32% after rejection of two corneal transplants and as little as 20% after rejection of three grafts [17]. Interestingly, there is a correlation between the onset and the severity of the rejection episode [15].

Size of a Corneal Graft
The diameter of a corneal graft contributes to the risk of graft failure. Many authors have demonstrated that engraftment of very large corneas results in an increased risk of graft rejection. The underlying explanation is that the larger a graft is, the more antigens that are carried into the host organism. In addition, the distance between the vascularized limbus and the allogeneic cornea is smaller compared to that for regular-sized grafts [22, 23].

Intraocular Surgery, Anterior Segment Inflammation
Surgical procedures performed simultaneously with or prior to pKP are associated with an increased risk of graft failure. Vitrectomy, lensectomy and surgical interventions to lower the eye pressure have been described as contributors to graft rejection, considering the fact that physiological processes in the anterior and/or posterior chamber are disrupted. Hence, anterior synechiae can increase the probability of graft failure by a factor of two if three or more quadrants are affected by iris adhesion [14, 24]. The underlying reason seems to be a loss of the immune privilege of the allogeneic graft [25]. However, shear forces

at the rear surface of the cornea may also lead to corneal endothelial cell loss [26]. An increase in eye pressure itself negatively affects the viability of the endothelium [26], thus resulting in expedited cell loss. Similarly, when pKP is performed in the acute state of anterior segment inflammation, the graft is prone to reduced survival. Unless not unavoidable (e.g. keratoplasty in emergency corneal perforations), such transplantation should be postponed for 6–12 months until a quiescent state of the anterior chamber is achieved [27].

Certain systemic diagnoses, such as Stevens-Johnson syndrome, ocular cicatricial pemphigoid, uveitis or atopic disease, render a bad prognosis for pKP. Such patients have be treated in an interdisciplinary fashion that may involve systemic immunosuppression. Open discussions with the patient are crucial to ensure cooperation after surgery.

Herpes Simplex
It has been widely accepted that keratitis caused by herpes simplex is a negative prognostic factor for pKP [28, 29]. The incidence of graft failure is significantly higher compared to that for conventional low-risk keratoplasties (e.g. in keratoconus); up to 70% of graft rejections are not reversible [30]. One reason for this high rate of irreversible graft failure might be the clinical similarity of regular graft failure and infection with herpes simplex virus [30]. Though the use of systemic antivirals for prophylaxis results in a reduction in herpes recurrence rates [26], pKPs after herpes simplex virus infection remain considerably threatened by immune rejection. In addition to the increased immunological risk, infected patients also suffer from neurotrophic disorders of the corneal surface, often resulting in impaired regeneration of the ocular surface.

Patient Age
The risk of corneal graft rejection increases with decreasing patient age. This is particularly evident in children, in whom the incidence of graft

failure within the first 2 years in patients younger than 15 years is as high as 30–40%. Compared to an older patient collective, patients below 40 years of age exhibit a risk of rejection that is twice as high as the risk of graft failure [31]. One reason for these difficulties may lie in the fact that younger donors express more HLAs, resulting in a higher probability of recognition of the graft by the host immune system [32].

Postoperative Management of High-Risk Keratoplasty

The treatment of high-risk keratoplasties requires specific attention to the topical and systemic application of therapeutics.

It is widely accepted that preservative-free topical antibiotics and lubricant should be administered until closure of the corneal epithelium. The use of steroids prior to epithelial wound closure is initially optional but is a necessity once an intact and stable epithelial layer is formed by the patient's corneal epithelial cells.

Treatment in Patients with Prior Herpes Simplex Infection
Prior to pKP, a prophylactic oral dose of 5 × 200 mg acyclovir per day is recommended. Postoperatively, this dose should be increased to oral 5 × 400 mg for the duration of the systemic steroid treatment [33, 34], with supportive topical acyclovir ointment.

Patients with an increased risk of recurrence of herpes simplex keratitis require daily dosages of 800–1,000 mg per day over 6–12 months [35, 36]. In cases with a high risk of immune rejection and herpes keratitis recurrence, mycophenolate mofetil (MMF) should be added at 2 × 1 g per day for 6–12 months [37].

Systemic steroids should be initially administered at a dosage of 1–2 mg/kg body weight per day and gradually tapered to achieve a total treatment period of around 3 weeks [38].

Systemic Treatment in High-Risk Settings and Human Leukocyte Antigen Matching

To enhance corneal graft survival in a high-risk environment, the basic steroid therapy described above has to be augmented by stronger immuno-suppressives (e.g. cyclosporin A, MMF). These replace corticosteroids in the mid-term and provide long-term immunosuppression.

In all cases of administration of systemic immunosuppressive drugs, a specialist in internal medicine has to be consulted to assess the overall risk of this form of immunosuppression. The liver, kidneys, blood and blood pressure have to be thoroughly examined because cyclosporin A can lead to hypertension and to nephrotoxicity and MMF can lead to hepatotoxicity and gastrointestinal problems.

Cyclosporin A is prescribed at a dose of 3–5 mg/kg body weight per day, with monitoring of the blood cyclosporin level (therapeutic level of 100–150 ng/ml; the level of the drug greatly varies between different laboratories and in relationship with the time of drug administration). The dosage has to be adapted according to the serum cyclosporin level. The duration of the treatment is determined by the individual graft rejection risk of the patient [39].

MMF can be applied in the presence of contraindications against cyclosporin A or in combination with acyclovir in the postoperative treatment of keratoplasties in patients suffering from herpes simplex keratitis. The recommended dose is 2 × 1 g per day. Choosing MMF as an immunosuppressive has the advantage of not requiring regular testing of the blood serum level.

An important approach propagated over the years is HLA matching of donors and recipients. Here, the patient's blood is examined for its HLA phenotype, which then is reported to large eye bank networks in an effort provide matching donor tissue as rapidly as possible. As donor tissues' HLA phenotype is also examined in certain eye banks, it is possible match a donor and a recipient. This increases the probability of reducing graft re-jection in high-risk keratoplasties [39]. Due to the changing indications of pKP in favor of lamellar keratoplasties (and especially Descemet's membrane endothelial keratoplasty (DMEK), with very low rejection rates), the earlier relevance of HLA typing is vanishing to a certain extent and is now limited to very high-risk re-pKP [40].

Risks of Lamellar Keratoplasty

The Role of Posterior Lamellar Keratoplasty

Since the development of new techniques for anterior and posterior lamellar surgery, layer-specific treatment of corneal pathologies has become feasible. While full-thickness keratoplasty was the gold standard for almost 100 years, the number of penetrating procedures is decreasing while the number of lamellar corneal surgeries is continuously increasing.

Endothelial pathologies, such as Fuchs' endothelial dystrophy, represent the majority of clinical cases in ophthalmological clinics in Europe and the Americas. Therefore, replacement of Descemet's membrane using Descemet's stripping automated endothelial keratoplasty (DSAEK) or DMEK is becoming predominant in ophthalmo-surgical routine practice [41].

As the corneal stroma and the corneal epithelium are considered to be the main carriers of the antigen load that triggers an immune response after engraftment, reduction in (in DSAEK) or elimination of (in DMEK) grafted stroma should subsequently result in a reduced immune reaction against the lamellar allograft. Indeed, Anshu and co-workers could demonstrate a 15-fold reduction in graft rejection in 1- and 2-year follow-ups for DSAEK versus pKP and even a 20-fold reduction when comparing DMEK to pKP in low-risk settings [42]. In DMEK, 1% of the cases demonstrated rejection episodes (at both 1 and 2 years), and in DSAEK, 8% and 12% did after 1 and 2 years, respectively. In contrast, pKP showed significantly higher rejections rates, or 14% and 18%, respectively [42].

Interestingly, the antigenic potency of DMEK grafts to induce a clinically relevant immune response by the host seems to be rather limited. It has been reported that a 10-fold reduction in the corticoid concentration (prednisolone acetate 1% vs. fluorometholone 0.1%) is still sufficient to maintain a rejection rate of 1% 1 year after DMEK transplantation [43].

The Role of Anterior Lamellar Keratoplasty

Anterior keratoplasty has generally been used as a partial substitute for pKP in indications with remaining physiological corneal endothelium (such as keratoconus or corneal scars) [44]. As the surgery itself is technically demanding and given that successful separation of Descemet's membrane from the stroma is a challenge, the number of surgeons performing conventional pKPs in these cases is still considerable [45].

In a meta-analysis, deep lamellar keratoplasty (DALK) and pKP were compared. As expected, the endothelial cell count in DALK cases was significantly higher, and the visual outcomes were better. The graft failure rate, however, and postoperative astigmatism were similar between the two groups. DALK patients showed fewer complications, e.g. no expulsive hemorragias or no endophthalmitis [46]. These findings, however, are controversial, as other authors detected no significant differences in a meta-analysis of DALK versus pKP for keratoconus [47]. Long-term data will clarify which surgical strategy is more beneficial for patients, considering both the risk of re-transplantation and the visual outcome.

Outlook

High-risk keratoplasties remain a considerable challenge for both surgical and conservative ophthalmologists. However, advances in immunosuppressives might open new strategies to prevent and treat allograft immune reactions in the future. The changing landscape of ophthalmosurgical reality – including the trend of replacing pKP with posterior lamellar keratoplasty in particular – represents a real breakthrough for patients. For certain indications, the risk of immune rejection following DMEK can be almost eradicated.

References

1 European Eye Bank Association, Venice, Italy, 2010.
2 Eye Bank Association of America, Washington DC, 2015.
3 Council on Scientific Affairs: Report on the organ transplant panel: corneal transplantation. JAMA 1988;259:719–722.
4 Mader TH, Stulting RD: The high-risk penetrating keratoplasty. Ophthalmol Clin North Am 1991;4:411–426.
5 Foulks GN, Sanfilippo F: Beneficial effects of histocompatibility on high-risk corneal transplantation. Am J Ophthalmol 1982;94:622–629.
6 Zirm EK: Eine erfolgreiche totale Keratoplastik. 1906 (A successful total keratoplasty). Refract Corneal Surg 1989;5: 258–261.
7 Paufique L, Sourdille GP, Offret G (eds): Les Graffes de la Cornée. Paris, Masson, 1948.
8 Maumenee AE: The influence of donor-recipient sensitization on corneal grafts. Am J Ophthalmol 1951;34:134–152.
9 Khodadoust AA, Silverstein AM: Transplantation and rejection of individual cell layers of the cornea. Invest Ophthalmol Vis Sci 1969;8:180–195.
10 Khodadoust AA, Silverstein AM: Studies on the nature of the privilege enjoyed by corneal allografts. Invest Ophthalmol Vis Sci 1972;11:137–148.
11 Klein J: Natural History of the Major Histocompatibility Complex. New York, Wiley, 1986.
12 Streilein JW: Immunobiology and immunopathology of corneal transplantation. Chem Immunol 1999;73:186–206.
13 Alldredge OC, Krachmer JH: Clinical types of corneal transplant rejection. Arch Ophthalmol 1981;99:599–604.
14 Maguire MG, Stark WJ, Gottsch JD, et al: Risk factors of corneal graft failure and rejection in the collaborative corneal transplantation studies. Collaborative Corneal Transplantation Studies Research Group. Ophthalmology 1994; 101:1536–1547.
15 The Collaborative Corneal Transplantation Studies Research Group: The collaborative corneal transplantation studies (CCTS). Effectiveness of histocompatibility matching in high-risk corneal transplantation. Arch Ophthalmol 1992;110:1392–1403.

16 Polack FM: Scanning electron microscopy of corneal graft rejection: epithelial rejection, endothelial rejection, and formation of posterior graft membranes. Invest Ophthalmol 1972;11:1–14.

17 Khodadoust AA: The allograft rejection reaction: the leading cause of late failure of clinical corneal grafts; in Jones BR (ed): Corneal Graft Failure. New York, Elsevier, 1972.

18 Fine M, Stein M: The role of corneal vascularization in human graft rejection; in Porter R, Knight J, Ciba Foundation (eds): Corneal Graft Failure. Amsterdam/New York, Associated Scientific Publishers, 1973, pp 193–204.

19 Nakamura S, Kinoshita S, Yokoi N, et al: Lacrimal hypofunction as a new mechanism of dry eye in visual display terminal users. PLoS One 2010;5:e11119.

20 Shimazaki J, Maruyama F, Shimmura S, et al: Immunologic rejection of the central graft after limbal allograft transplantation combined with penetrating keratoplasty. Cornea 2001;20:149–152.

21 Reinhard T, Spelsberg H, Henke L, et al: Long-term results of allogeneic penetrating limbo-keratoplasty in total limbal stem cell deficiency. Ophthalmology 2004;111:775–782.

22 Boisjoly HM, Bernard PM, Dube I, et al: Effects of factors unrelated to tissue matching on corneal transplant endothelial rejection. Am J Ophthalmol 1989; 107:647–654.

23 Volker-Dieben HJ, D'Amaro J, Kok-van Alphen CC: Hierarchy of prognostic factors for corneal allograft survival, Aust N Z J Ophthalmol 1987;15:11–18.

24 Sit M, Weisbrod DJ, Noar J, et al: Corneal graft outcome study. Cornea 2001; 20:129–133.

25 Yamagami S, Tsuru T: Increase in orthotopic murine corneal transplantation rejection rate with anterior synechiae. Invest Ophthalmol Vis Sci 1999;40: 2422–2426.

26 Wilson SE, Kaufman HE: Graft failure after penetrating keratoplasty. Surv Ophthalmol 1990;34:325–356.

27 Nobe JR, Moura BT, Robin JB, et al: Results of penetrating keratoplasty for the treatment of corneal perforations. Arch Ophthalmol 1990;108:939–941.

28 Coster DJ: Factors affecting the outcome of corneal transplantation. Ann R Coll Surg Engl 1981;63:91–97.

29 Moyes AL, Sugar A, Musch DC, et al: Antiviral therapy after penetrating keratoplasty for herpes simplex keratitis. Arch Ophthalmol 1994;112:601–607.

30 Epstein RJ, Seedor JA, Dreizen NG, et al: Penetrating keratoplasty for herpes simplex keratitis and keratokonus. Allograft rejection and survival. Ophthalmology 1987;94:935–944.

31 Stulting RD, Sumers KD, Cavanagh HD, et al: Penetrating keratoplasty in children. Ophthalmology 1984;91:1222–1230.

32 Palay DA, Kangas TA, Stulting RD, et al: The effects of donor age on the outcome of penetrating keratoplasty in adults. Ophthalmology 1997;104:1576–1579.

33 Barney NP, Foster CS: A prospective randomized trial of oral acyclovir after penetrating keratoplasty for herpes simplex keratitis. Cornea 1994;13:232–236.

34 Kersten A, Sundmacher R, Reinhard T: Postoperative Komplikationen nach perforierender Keratoplastik in Herpesaugen. Differentialdiagnose, Therapie und prognostische Bedeutung. Ophthalmologe 1997;94:889–896.

35 Tambasco FP, Cohen EJ, Nguyen LH, et al: Oral Acyclovir after penetrating keratoplasty for herpes simplex keratitis. Arch Ophthalmol 1999;117:445–449.

36 van Rooij J, Rijneveld WJ, Remeijer L, et al: Effect of oral acyclovir after penetrating keratoplasty for herpetic keratitis: a placebo-controlled multicenter trial. Ophthalmology 2003;110:1916–1919.

37 Mayer K, Reinhard T, Reis A, et al: Synergistic antiherpetic effect of acyclovir and mycofenolate mofetil following keratoplasty in patients with herpetic eye disease: first results of a randomized püilot study. Graefe's Arch Clin Exp Ophthalmol 2003;214:1051–1054.

38 Hill JC: Immunosuppression in corneal transplantation. Eye 1995;9:247–253.

39 Reinhard T, Sundmacher R, Godehardt E, et al: Systemische Cyclosporin-A-Prophylaxe nach Keratoplastiken mit erhöhtem Risiko für Immunreaktionen als einzigem erhöhten Risikofaktor. Ophthalmologe 1997;94:496–500.

40 Böhringer D, Ihorst G, Grotejohann B, et al: Functional antigen matching in corneal transplantation: matching for the HLA-A, -B and -DRB1 antigens (FANCY) – study protocol. BMC Ophthalmol 2014;14:156.

41 Rodríguez-Calvo-de-Mora M, Quilendrino R, Ham L, et al: Clinical outcome of 500 consecutive cases undergoing Descemet's membrane endothelial keratoplasty. Ophthalmology 2015;122:464–470.

42 Anshu A, Price MO, Price FW Jr: Risk of corneal transplant rejection significantly reduced with Descemet's membrane endothelial keratoplasty. Ophthalmology 2012;119:536–540.

43 Price MO, Price FW Jr, Kruse FE, et al: Randomized comparison of topical prednisolone acetate 1% versus fluorometholone 0.1% in the first year after descemet membrane endothelial keratoplasty. Cornea 2014;33:880–886.

44 Sarnicola V, Toro P, Sarnicola C, et al: Long-term graft survival in deep anterior lamellar keratoplasty. Cornea 2012; 31:621–626.

45 Kasbekar SA, Jones MN, Ahmad S, et al: Corneal transplant surgery for keratoconus and the effect of surgeon experience on deep anterior lamellar keratoplasty outcomes. Am J Ophthalmol 2014;158: 1239–1246.

46 Liu H, Chen Y, Wang P, et al: Efficacy and safety of deep anterior lamellar keratoplasty vs. penetrating keratoplasty for keratoconus: a meta-analysis. PLoS One 2015;10:e0113332.

47 Keane M, Coster D, Ziaei M, et al: Deep anterior lamellar keratoplasty versus penetrating keratoplasty for treating keratoconus. Cochrane Database Syst Rev 2014;7:CD009700.

Prof. Dr. med. Friedrich E. Kruse
Department of Ophthalmology
University of Erlangen-Nürnberg
Schwabachanlage 6
DE–91054 Erlangen (Germany)
E-Mail friedrich.kruse@uk-erlangen.de

Güell JL (ed): Cornea. ESASO Course Series. Basel, Karger, 2015, vol 6, pp 81–101
DOI: 10.1159/000381495

Deep Anterior Lamellar Keratoplasty: Surgical Technique, Indications, Clinical Results and Complications

Enrica Sarnicola[a] · Caterina Sarnicola[b] · Vincenzo Sarnicola[c]

[a]University of Siena, Siena, [b]University of Ferrara, Ferrara, and [c]Ambulatorio di Chirurgia Oculare 'Santa Lucia', Grosseto, Italy

Abstract

Deep anterior lamellar keratoplasty (DALK) is currently the procedure of choice to restore transparency and curvature in corneal stromal diseases with a healthy endothelium. Preserving the endothelium avoids endothelial rejection and provides a good and stable endothelial cell count, allowing good long-term graft survival. Several surgical techniques have been proposed over the last years, the most common of which include layer-by-layer manual dissection, hydrodissection, viscodissection, big bubble (needle or cannula) and air-viscobubble. Descemet's membrane rupture represents the most common complication, even in expert hands. The penetrating keratoplasty conversion rate gradually decreases as surgeons become more experienced and learn to manage Descemet's membrane ruptures. Being able to repair the ruptures would increase the success of DALK and allow patients to benefit from all of its advantages.

© 2015 S. Karger AG, Basel

Introduction

In the last 15 years, corneal transplantation has moved from a full-thickness transplant approach (penetrating keratoplasty (PK)) to a selective and minimally invasive approach in which only the diseased portions of the cornea are replaced and the healthy layers are preserved (lamellar keratoplasty (LK)).

Limbal stem cell transplantation (conjunctival limbal autograft, living-related conjunctival limbal allograft, keratolimbal allograft, combined conjunctival limbal and keratolimbal allograft, cultivated limbal epithelial transplantation, or cultivated oral mucosal epithelial transplantation), which is the proper treatment for ocular surface transplantation, aims to restore self-maintenance and self-regeneration of the epithelia for defense against external insults. Anterior LK (superficial anterior LK (SALK), deep anterior LK (DALK), etc.) represents the treatment of choice for stromal corneal diseases that do not affect the endothelium. Analogously, posterior LK (deep lamellar endothelial keratoplasty (DLEK), Descemet's stripping endothelial keratoplasty (DSEK), Descemet's stripping automated endothelial keratoplasty (DSAEK), or Descemet's membrane endothelial keratoplasty (DMEK)) is the proper approach for the treatment of endothelial diseases.

DALK, which allowing for a total or subtotal replacement of the stroma and leaving the recipi-

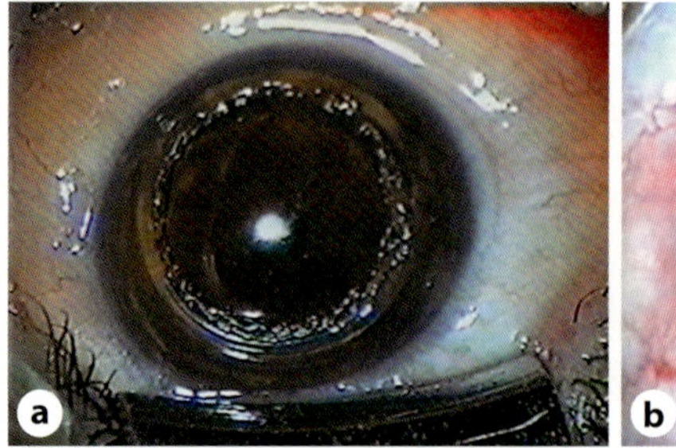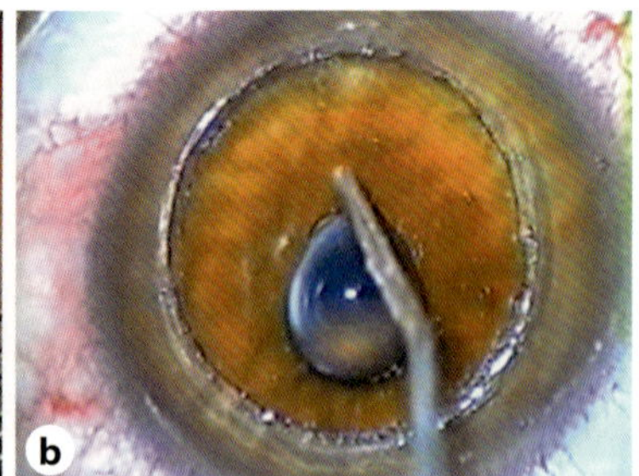

Fig. 1. Descemet's membrane (DM) exposure. **a** DM exposure (dDALK); **b** predescemetic plane exposure (pdDALK).

ent Descemet's membrane (DM) and endothelium intact, has been a fundamental change in recent years.

Surgical Techniques

History

Although the validity of a lamellar corneal transplantation was originally proposed by von Hipple in 1888 [1], LK involved a time-consuming and difficult free-hand dissection that produced interface irregularities, usually resulting in the loss of vision, or only partial improvements. Given the difficulty of achieving good visual outcomes, PK, no matter what kind of corneal disease, has represented the mainstay of corneal transplantation surgery since the mid-1950s, until recently, thanks to the introduction of topical steroids [2].

Advances in technology and techniques, as well as a greater understanding of corneal physiology and optics, facilitated the resumption of lamellar surgery. In 1971, José Barraquer outlined the necessary rules to accomplish good visual results with LK: 1) trying to obtain the deepest possible interface to reduce scarring, 2) attaining a posterior layer of uniform thickness, 3) performing a smooth surface sectioning of both the graft and the bed, 4) cutting the graft of the appropriate thickness, 5) using the highest quality donor material, 6) insuring a good coaptation of the edges and uniform traction of the sutures, and make sure that there is perfect

cleanliness of the interface [3]. It is now clear that José Barraquer was referring to the features of what would have been later called predecemetic DALK (pdDALK).

It is critical to understand what is intended by the terms descemetic DALK (dDALK) and pdDALK. In dDALK all of the host stroma is removed, and only the DM and the endothelium are preserved. José Barraquer's rules are not so important for this approach because DM is already smooth, regular and uniform in thickness (fig. 1a).

Conversely pdDALK results when the surgeon, in an attempt to expose the DM, fails in this purpose and leaves a thin layer of stroma over the DM and the endothelium. This usually occurs with manual dissection (layer-by-layer) technique [4] (fig. 1b).

The literature shows how manual stromectomy has left room for other techniques that actually allow for an easier separation of stroma and DM. In 1997, Sugita and Kondo [5] suggested the injection of balanced salt solution into the stroma (hydrodissection). In 1999, Melles et al. [6, 7] described the use of viscoelastic materials (viscodissection). Air dissection was proposed by Anwar in 1972 [8] and was later modified by Archila in 1985 [9], Price in 1989 [10] and Chau et al. in 1992 [11], and finally its 'big bubble' (BB) variant was designed by Anwar and Teichmann in 2002 [12].

Currently, the DALK techniques most commonly used are the following:
– Layer-by-layer manual dissection
– Hydrodissection

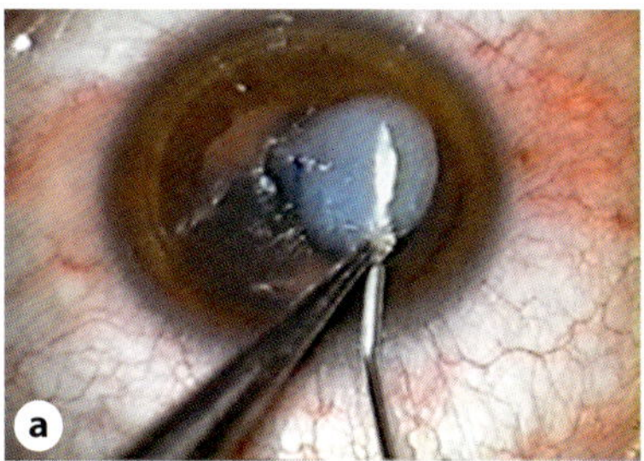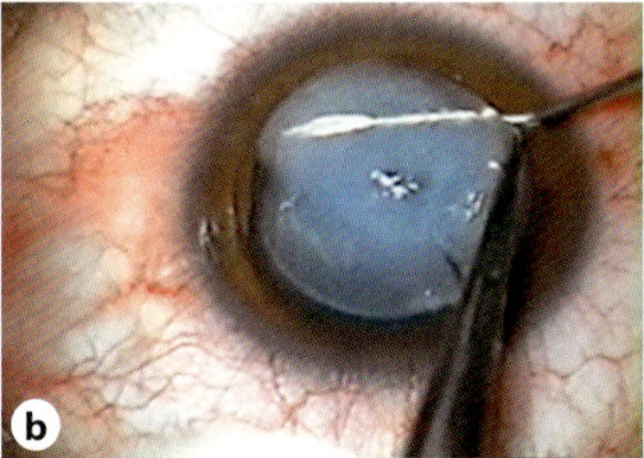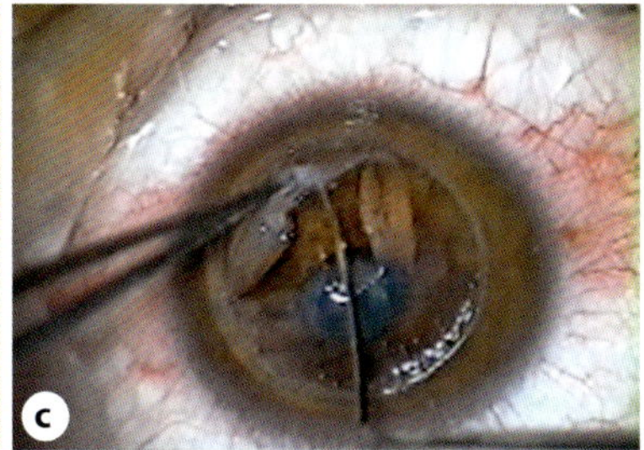

Fig. 2. Hydrodissection (**a**). A 27 gauge needle attached to a balanced salt solution-filled syringe is inserted into the corneal stroma after anterior lamellar keratectomy; **b** balanced salt solution progression detaches DM from the stroma. Collagen fibers become white and swollen; **c** stromal removal via spatula-mediated delamination.

– Viscoelastic dissection
– Air BB
– Air-viscobubble (AVB)

Stromal Dissection

Layer-by-Layer Manual Dissection

Dry manual layer-by-layer dissection is probably the oldest technique of LK, which regained prominence when Tsubota et al. [13] applied the principles of '*divide-and-conquer*' from cataract surgery. After trephination, the recipient cornea is divided into four quadrants to facilitate lamellar dissection at a depth of approximately 70%. This procedure of division is continued until the central area (about 5 mm in diameter) of DM is exposed. The authors reported almost 6% of DM ruptures, which were repaired by injecting air into the anterior chamber.

Hydrodissection

This technique was first described by Sugita and Kondo in 1997 [5]. Firstly, a trephine blade is turned downward through the cornea until three quarters of its depth, and then, a lamellar keratectomy is performed with a Golf or Paufique knife. The cut is made with the blade moving as if stroking this area. A small cut/depression is created in the deeper stroma. A 27-gauge needle attached to a syringe is inserted at the bottom of the depres-

sion, and balanced salt solution is injected into the stromal bed (fig. 2a). The solution penetrates into the collagen fibers, which whiten and swell and which can be safely removed by further delamination (using a spatula, forceps and scissors) (fig. 2b, c). As DM is approached, it bulges forward and can be recognized by its shiny, smooth appearance. Perforations are common at this stage (39.2% in this study) and can be managed by air injection into anterior chamber.

Viscodissection

Melles et al., in 1999, described a technique that uses ophthalmic viscoelastic device (OVD) injection to separate DM from the stroma. A 30 gauge needle attached to a viscoelastic material-filled syringe is inserted into the corneal stroma as close to DM as possible. To visualize the depth of corneal incision and lamellar dissection during surgery, they created an air-to-endothelium interface that behaves as a convex mirror, by exchanging the aqueous space of the anterior chamber with air [6]. The non reflective dark bend, seen between the balde tip and the light reflex, represents the nonincised corneal tissue between the blade and the air-to-endothelium interface. Since the dark band becomes thinner by advancing of the blade into the deeper stromal layers, the corneal depth of the blade can be judged by the thickness of the dark band. When the tip of the needle appears to touch the light reflex (the posterior

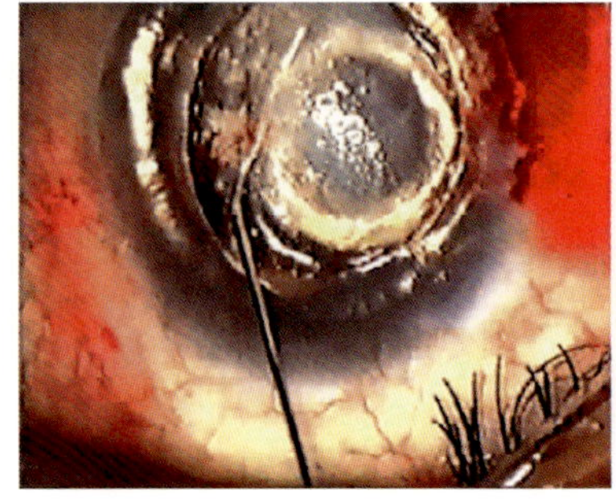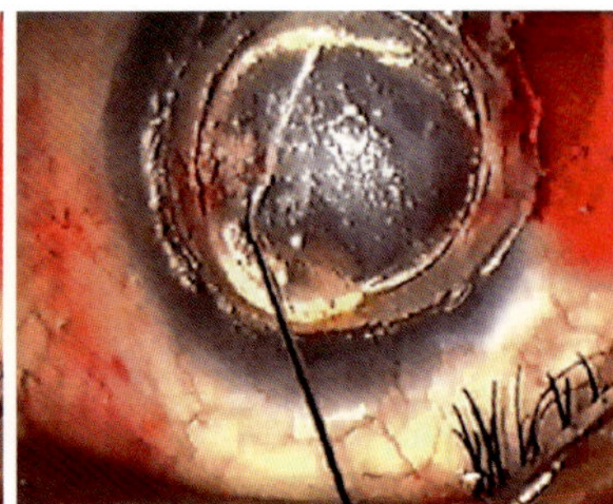

Fig. 3. Viscodissection. 'Golden ring' reflex outlines the progression wave of ophthalmic viscoelastic device (OVD) between DM and the stroma.

corneal surface), an OVD can be injected into the cornea to separate DM from the overlying posterior stroma. The progression of the OVD between these two layers is outlined by a typical reflex (we call it a 'golden ring' [4] (fig. 3)). After a corneal pocket filled with the OVD is created, a suction trephine is centered over the anterior corneal surface. The blade is turned downward until viscoelastic material is seen to escape from the pocket through the trephine incision. The stroma over the pocket is excised, and the recipient bed is thoroughly irrigated to remove all of the OVD and debris [14].

Although this technique provides good results, it is not always easy to identify the reflex.

Needle Big Bubble
The BB technique, originally described by Anwar and Teichmann in 2002 [12], is the most used DALK procedure. According to a study by Sarnicola et al., BB provides the highest rate of DM exposure [4]. In a major review of lamellar corneal transplantation, Arenas et al. stated that the BB technique 'is a faster and reliable way of baring the DM' [15]. A suction trephine is used to perform a partial thickness corneal trephination at a depth of about 60–80%. A 27- or 30-gauge needle attached to an air-filled syringe is inserted deep into the paracentral stroma through the bottom of the trephination groove and is advanced so that the bevel remains parallel to DM and faces down. At this point, air is injected, forming a large air bubble between DM and the corneal stroma in

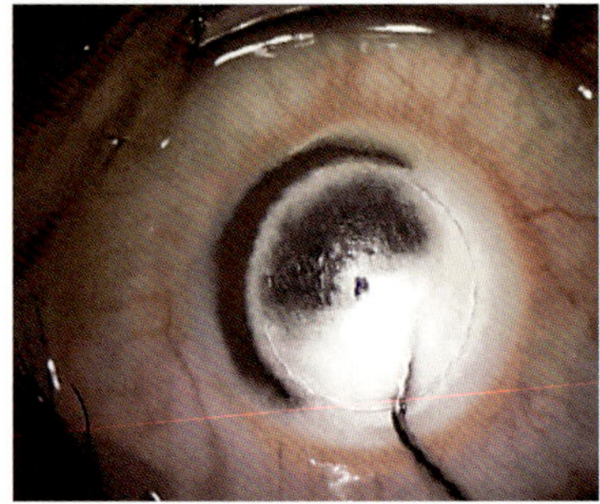

Fig. 4. Anwar needle-based big bubble (BB) technique: BB formation.

most cases (60–70%) (fig. 4). After performing an anterior keratectomy, a small opening in the center of the anterior wall of the bubble is made. This step should be performed using a sharp tip of a pointed blade held almost parallel to the surface. Collapse of the air bubble then occurs, and the knife is quickly withdrawn (fig. 5). The remaining stromal layers are lifted with an iris spatula, severed with a blade, and excised with scissors [12].

The BB opening technique has been refined by Goshe et al. [16] who proposed to coat the overlying stroma with cohesive viscoelastic material prior to entering the BB. A 1.0–1.5 mm incision is then created with a 1.0 mm diamond knife using only the tip of the blade through a 'lifting' motion. Goshe et al. reports two advantages of this opening technique. First, when the stroma is incised to enter the BB, little to no air escapes from the bubble. This prevents a sudden collapse of the bubble, which can cause the blade to perforate DM. Sec-

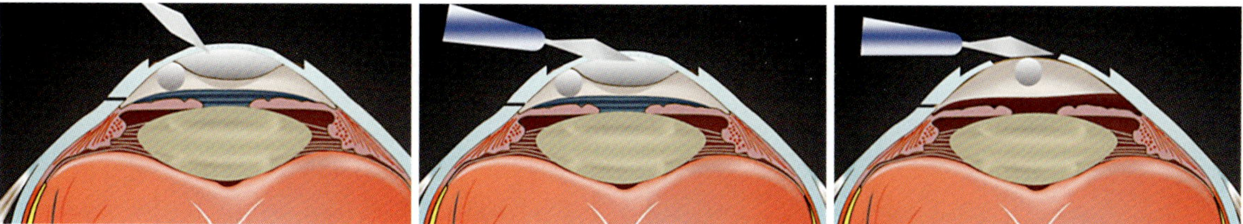

Fig. 5. Anwar needle-based BB opening. When the BB is open, DM changes shape from concave to convex upward. At the same time, the small air bubble in the anterior chamber moves from the periphery toward the center (the bubble test becomes negative).

Fig. 6. New BB opening. **a** BB covered by an OVD; **b** opening of the bubble with a cut made from the bottom upward using a cataract knife.

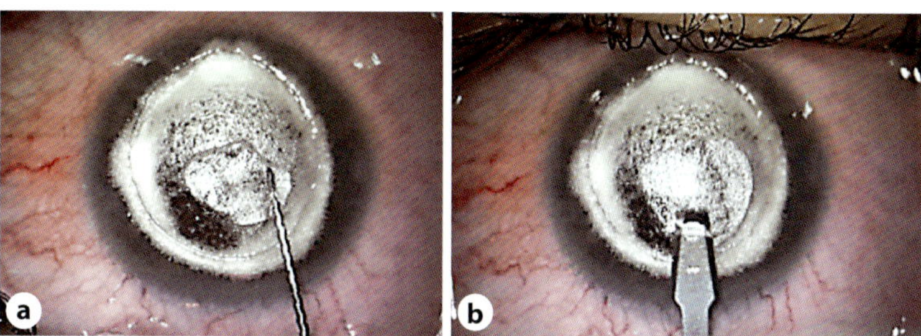

ond, an air-viscoelastic material exchange can be performed to maintain space in the bubble to facilitate the sweeping of the peripheral interface and the subsequent resection of the residual cap.

Our modification [unpublished data, presented at the American Academy of Ophthalmology annual meeting in 2011] of this new opening of the bubble involves the use of a cataract knife. After covering the corneal surface with an OVD, a cut is made through a bottom-up movement of the knife. This kind of cut provides the advantage of further limiting the release of air from the bubble. Then, OVD is injected inside the bubble to create a safe space between the stroma and DM so that corneal stroma removal can be performed with less risks (fig. 6).

Sometimes, the air injection can cause corneal emphysema. In such cases, the whitening of the cornea prevents the discernment of whether the BB has been successfully achieved. Parthasarathy et al. [17] described a technique for immediately determining the formation of the bubble, which we like to call the 'bubble test'. A small air bubble is injected into the anterior chamber via a limbal paracentesis. If the small air bubble is then seen at the periphery of the anterior chamber, the separation of DM, induced by the BB, will be confirmed to have been successfully accomplished, as the convexity of the bubble will protrude posteriorly, forcing the small anterior chamber bubble to the periphery (fig. 7). If the small anterior chamber bubble is not seen in the anterior chamber periphery, it will mean that it is located centrally beneath the opaque corneal stroma and, therefore, that no BB has been produced (fig. 5).

Cannula Big Bubble
The use of a special blunt cannula [18–20] has been proposed to let surgeons go as deep as possible into the corneal stroma, without being afraid of DM perforation as when using a pointed instrument. It is common opinion that the deeper the air is injected, the higher the chances of generating a BB. Sarnicola and Toro described the surgical steps for achieving a BB using a blunt cannula [21] (fig. 8). These are similar to those previously de-

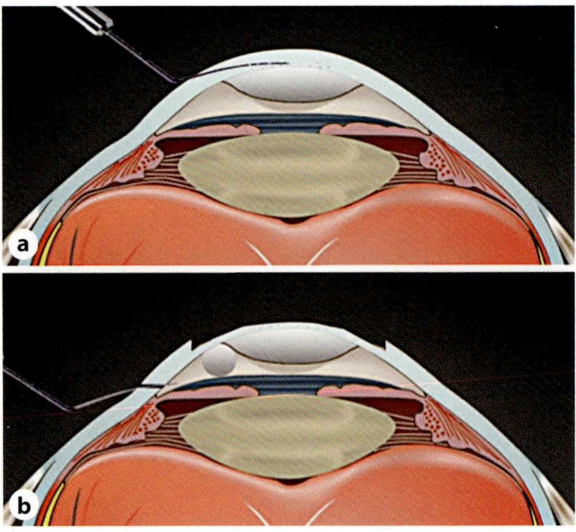

Fig. 7. Positive bubble test. **a** Successful BB formation: DM is concave upward; **b** positive bubble test: a small air bubble injected into the anterior chamber remains in the periphery.

scribed for obtaining a BB using a needle, except for two important modifications. After a partial corneal trephination, a smooth spatula (fig. 9a) is inserted as deep as possible into the peripheral trephination groove. The spatula is moved forward in the attempt to reach the predescemetic plane, deeper and deeper toward the center of the cornea. Once the predescemetic plane is reached, two important signs are frequently observed: reduced resistance of the advancement of the spatula and the appearance of DM folds. The spatula can then be removed, leaving a corneal tunnel into which a 27-gauge cannula attached to a 5cc air-filled syringe is inserted (fig. 9b). The cannula has a port that faces down so that air can push DM posteriorly. After advancing the cannula to the center of the cornea, air can be injected.

The literature shows that using a cannula to inject air provides the highest rate of successful BB accomplishment. Fourniè et al. indicated a BB success rate of 76.9% in a study of 13 eyes [22]. Sarnicola and Toro reported BB formation in 86% of cases in a study of 28 eyes [21].

Air-Viscobubble Dissection

AVB is a technique designed to manage those cases in which BB formation has failed (fig. 10). When air dissection does not result in big-bubble formation, superficial keratectomy is performed with a Golf knife. A new deeper tunnel is created into the stroma using the same spatula. The same cannula used for the air injection is then attached to a viscoelastic material-filled syringe, and viscodissection is tried as a second approach to separate DM from the corneal stroma. Sarnicola et al. reported the percentage of dDALK obtained with this combined technique: AVB helped to attain dDALK dissection in 7% of cases that together with the 86% of cases in which dDALK dissection had been achieved with the BB technique using a cannula, resulted in a total achievement of dDALK in 93% of cases [21].

The AVB technique of Sarnicola was studied in vitro by Muftuoglu et al. [23]. They evaluated the corneas after the failure of air BB formation using anterior segment optical coherence tomography and histopathologic examinations. They found small detachments in those cases when air BB was not achieved. They postulated that the additional OVD injection enabled dDALK dissection by building up the pressure inside the small bubbles upto spontaneous coalescence, thereby forming a large DM detachment.

In summary, in our experience, the introduction of the cannula BB and AVB techniques allowed for an increase in the rate of dDALK (separation of DM from the stroma) from 60% of cases using the Anwar needle-based BB technique to 93% of cases.

Donor Preparation

The donor corneal lenticule is usually punched on the endothelial side. DM has to be gently stripped off the donor cornea using a dry triangular swab or, even better, with forceps. Trypan blue

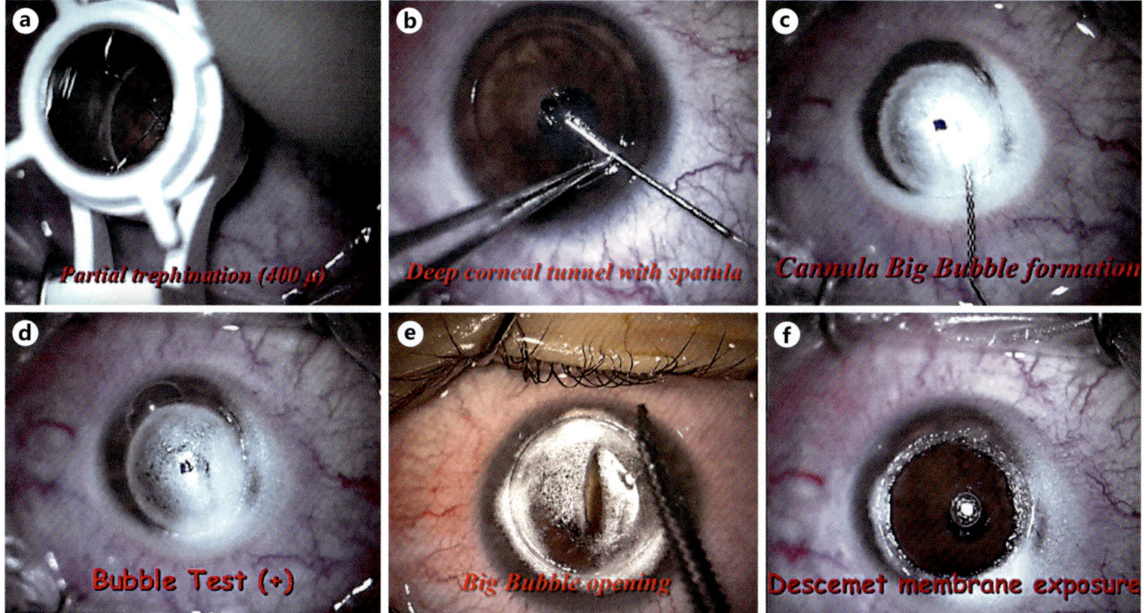

Fig. 8. a–f Surgical steps for cannula BB technique.

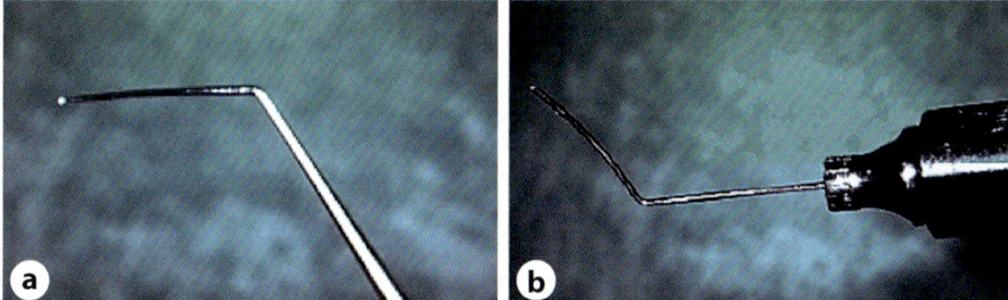

Fig. 9. a Sarnicola smooth spatula; **b** Sarnicola blunt cannula.

dye can be used to stain DM, especially when the endothelium is damaged with a swab (fig. 11).

Most of the studies published in literature show that the diameter of the donor cornea generally oversizes the recipient by 0.25 mm. Nonetheless other authors suggested the use of equivalent diameters [24] in order to reduce postoperative myopia: we personally agree with this approach. The use of a smaller-sized graft is still a matter of discussion. It could help to reduce postoperative myopia, but it has also been associated with a higher risk of DM wrinkles. However, wrinkles become less visible and may completely disappear over time. We suggest the use of a smaller-sized graft when anisometropia greater than 3 D myopic is present in the eye to operate. Moreover, a smaller donor cannot be used if a DM rupture occurs during stromectomy, because the disparity of curvature between the donor and the recipient prevents the management of DM rupture.

Suturing Techniques

Which suturing technique is the best still represents a controversial topic. Some surgeons support continuous sutures, whereas others are in

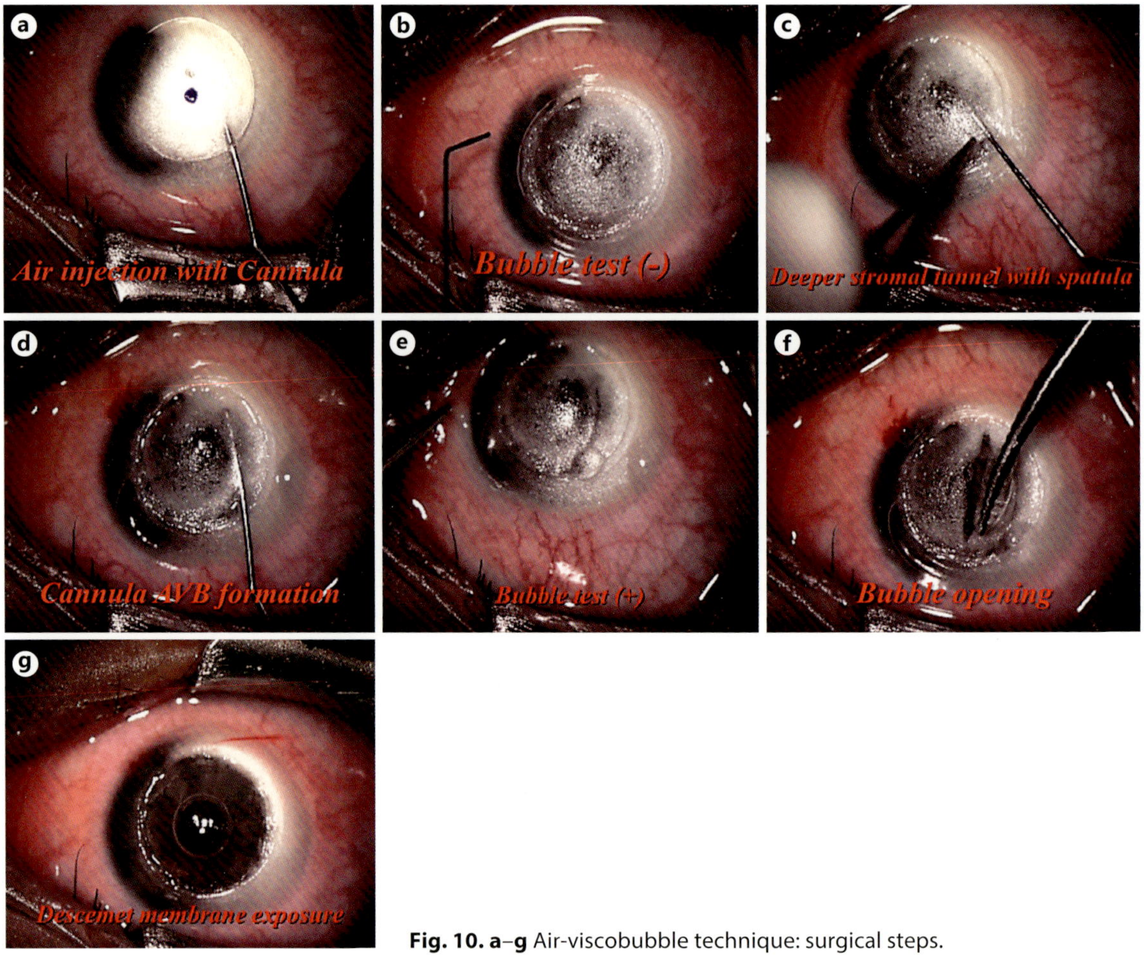

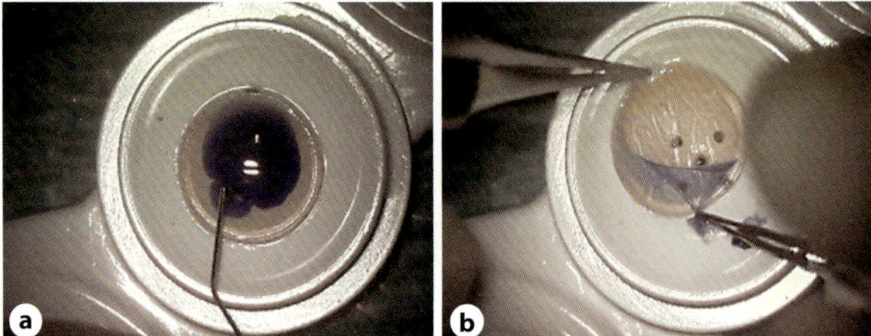

Fig. 10. a–g Air-viscobubble technique: surgical steps.

Fig. 11. Donor preparation. **a** DM staining with Trypan blue dye; **b** DM stripping using forceps.

favor of interrupted sutures. However, interrupted sutures have some evident advantages, such as easier management of postoperative astigmatism and DM ruptures (described in the Complications section).

New Devices

The use of Femtosecond laser trephination, combined with the BB or Melles technique, seems to be valuable in reducing postoperative astigmatism,

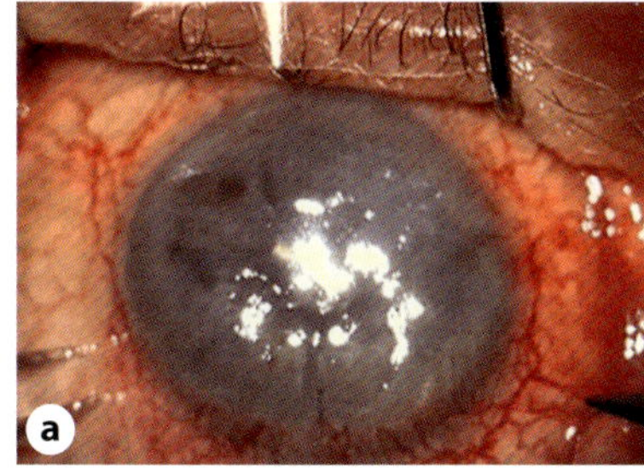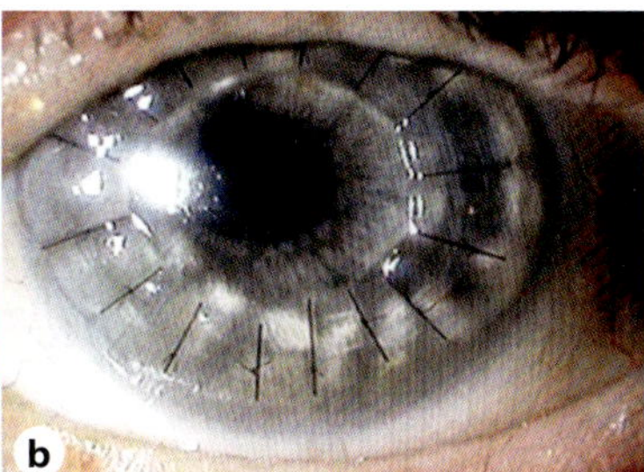

Fig. 12. Deep anterior lamellar keratoplasty (DALK) for Fusarium keratitis. **a** Preoperative; **b** postoperative.

improving wound healing, and allowing for earlier suture removal. This device helps in the construction of 'zig-zag' and 'mushroom' wounds in both the recipient and donor [25–30]. Nonetheless femtosecond lasers do not seem to be able to create very deep lamellar stromal cuts or to leave a uniform thickness of the recipient bed: two very important conditions for good visual recovery.

Preoperative and intraoperative imaging devices such as optical coherence tomography (OCT) and pachymetry can be used to increase the rate of dDALK [31–34].

Indications

Since the evolution of surgical techniques enabled good visual outcomes comparable to those of PK, DALK has become the gold standard technique to treat all diseases affecting the corneal stroma. Requiring healthy endothelium is the only restriction.

The graft remains clear thanks to the endothelial pump function, which is related to good endothelial cell density (ECD). ECD, continuing to drop for many years after PK surgery, can result in functional exhaustion. With DALK, given that the healthy host endothelium is not replaced, the ECD remains stable. It is easy to understand why young people affected by stromal pathologies may greatly benefit from DALK. For this reason, keratoconus has become the most common DALK indication in the last 15 years [35–39]. The corneal dystrophies [40–44] not involving the en-

dothelium and mucopolysaccharidosis [44, 45] (which usually affects infants) have also been treated with DALK and have shown good results.

Another major advantage of DALK is that endothelial rejection cannot occur. Epithelial, subepithelial and stromal rejection can still happen, but they are easily treatable using steroid eye drops most of the time. This is crucial for those pathologies associated with a high risk of rejection, like extreme ectatic disorders that require a large transplant. The proximity of the donor graft and the recipient limbus is responsible for a very high risk of immunological response [15, 37, 46]. Infectious stromal keratitis unresponsive to medical treatment is often characterized by inflammation and corneal neovascularization. In these cases, early therapeutic DALK not only avoids endothelial rejection and failure, but also limits the intraocular spread of the infection [15, 47–49, data under peer review for publication, presented at the VII World Cornea Congress, San Diego 2015, 'Precocious DALK in active keratitis poorly responsive to medical treatment'] (fig. 12, 13).

The relationship between rejection and recurrence of the infection is particularly true in herpes simplex virus infection. Rejection can cause recurrence of the infection and *vice versa*. DALK reduces immunological issues because the host endothelium is not replaced. Preoperative long-term therapy with oral acyclovir 800 mg/day, along with steroid eye drops once a day, and a postoperative prophylactic protocol prevented

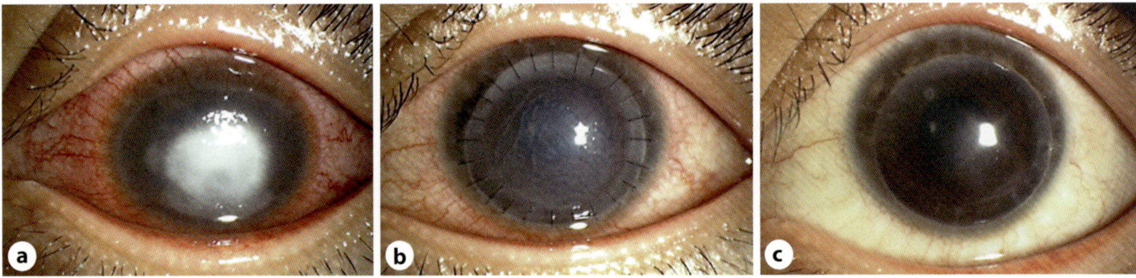

Fig. 13. DALK for *Acanthamoeba* keratitis. **a** Preoperative; **b** immediate postoperative. The corneal graft is centered on the infection site. **c** One year postoperative.

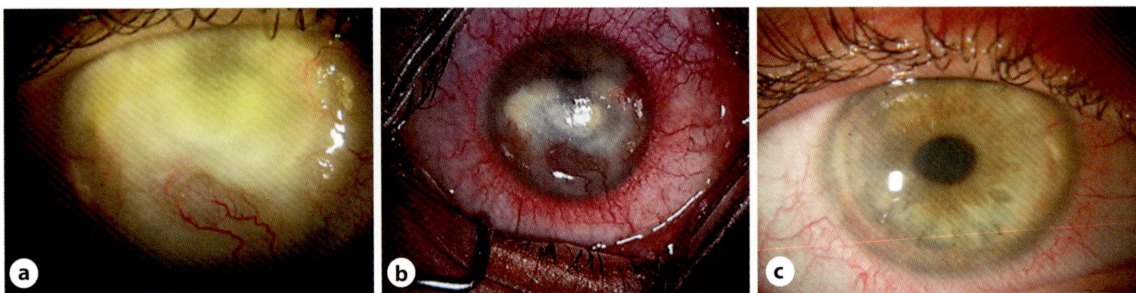

Fig. 14. DALK for herpes simplex virus infection. **a** Misdiagnosed herpes simplex virus infection; **b** preoperative: reduction of the central leucoma 6 months after oral acyclovir and topical steroid therapy; **c** 1 year postoperatively.

the recurrence of infection. Following this approach, no episodes of rejection or graft failure were observed in one of the largest case series of DALK performed for post-herpetic corneal stromal scarring (fig. 14). The postoperative treatment protocol consisted of both topical antibiotics and corticosteroids 4 times a day, along with oral acyclovir (800 mg) 3 times a day for the first month. During the second month, the regimen had been changed to dexamethasone eye drops (3 times a day) together with oral acyclovir 800 mg twice daily. After this point, long-term therapy consisted of oral acyclovir 800 mg once a day and loteprednol etabonate eye drops twice daily [50]. Several other studies [51–54] reported that DALK represents a good treatment for postherpetic stromal scarring. The postoperative prophylactic treatment was shorter, and this might probably be the reason why a certain percentage of recurrence has been reported in these studies.

However, DALK was shown to result in lower recurrence and rejection rates, and a higher graft survival rate than PK.

In summary, the following is a list of DALK indications.

– Corneal ectasia (keratoconus, keratoglobus, post-laser-assisted in situ keratomileusis ectasia [15, 55–57], pellucid marginal degeneration, recurrence of ectasia in previous PK [58, 59], etc.)
– Corneal stromal dystrophies when the endothelium is not affected (macular corneal dystrophy, granular corneal dystrophy, lattice corneal dystrophy and Avellino dystrophy)
– Corneal scarring (secondary to trauma, infection, chemical injury [15, 60, 61], mucopolysaccharidosis, etc.)
– Infectious stromal keratitis unresponsive to medical treatment (fungi, bacteria, or *Acanthamoeba*)

- Corneal melting (autoimmune, neurotrophic or infectious) [35]
- Descemetoceles [35, 62–64]
- Penetrating corneal wound without loss of substance [65, data under peer review for publication, presented at the XX Congreso Argentino de Oftalmologia, Buenos Aires 2015, 'pdDALK in corneal penetrating wounds']

Clinical Results

Visual Acuity

No significant difference in best spectacles-corrected VA (BSCVA) between DALK and PK has been found [35, 36]. According to the data from different studies, BSCVA after DALK ranges from 20/40 to 20/20 (49% of cases in one study and 64.3% in another study) [38, 66].

Conflicting opinions have arisen regarding BSCVA after dDALK or pdDALK. Sarnicola et al. studied BSCVA after DALK in 120 eyes. Sixty-one eyes were dDALK, and fifty-nine eyes were pdDALK. Visual outcomes were not significantly different between dDALK and pdDALK, although visual recovery was slightly delayed in the latter group. At the 30.4 months follow-up, BSCVA in the dDALK group was 20/30 or better in 85% of cases and was 20/20 in 49% of cases, and BSCVA in the pdDALK group was 20/30 or better in 80% of cases and was 20/20 in 49% of cases. The mean BSCVA was 0.88 in the dDALK group and 0.86 in the pdDALK group (p = 0.40) [38]. Bhatt et al. also compared visual outcomes obtained with the BB technique and the manual dissection technique (it can be supposed that this method is a pdDALK technique: '…manual lamellar dissection of stroma to get as close to the DM as possible') among 46 patients. There were no significant differences in BSCVA, astigmatism, contrast sensivity or densitometry in the two groups [67].

Another study reported that visual recovery from pdDALK was worse than that from dDALK. Fontana et al. compared BSCVA between three groups: PK (22 patients), dDALK (28 patients), and pdDALK (32 patients). In their study, the quality of vision after DALK was comparable to that after PK when dDALK was achieved, but was worse than that after PK when layers of the stroma had been left adherent to DM. The percentage of eyes with 20/20 BSCVA or better was 4 times higher in the PK and dDALK eyes than in the pdDALK eyes [68].

Analyzing these data the question that might arise could be, does pdDALK produce comparable visual results to those of dDALK? Why have these differences been observed in the literature?

The first thing to notice is that the residual host bed thickness has not reported in any of the cited studies. The study, following discussed, can help to answer our questions.

A precise explanation of what is intended with pdDALK is probably the key for interpreting the different results mentioned above. How much stroma can be left in the recipient bed to achieve good VA? Some authors clarified this issue. Ardjomand et al. reported that eyes with a recipient corneal bed thickness <20 μm had VA comparable with those receiving PK, whereas eyes with a thicker recipient corneal bed, >80 μm, had significantly reduced VA [69]. Reinhart et al., reviewing the published literature regarding DALK, reported that 'There was no significant difference in postoperative VA between DALK or PK eyes as a group, although there was a tendency for lower VA in DALK eyes in which DM was not bared and residual stroma in the bed exceeded 10% of total stromal thickness' [36].

We can say that Ardjomand answered to our questions. The term pdDALK was probably used to indicate all cases in which a layer-by-layer delamination technique had been performed, regardless of the depth of the dissection. Some surgeons go deeper than others. It might be the case that, in order to effectively analyze an homogenous group of results, only DALK with a residual bed thickness <80 μm should be called pdDALK. *'Indeed, this surgery is named deep anterior lamellar keratoplasty, so…it is very important how deep is the surgeon'.*

Endothelial Cell Density

Good postoperative ECD is one of the most important features in favor of DALK. All of the published studies show that endothelial cell loss (ECL) is significantly lower with DALK rather than with PK [2, 35–37]. In a retrospective study with the longest follow-up duration (6 months to 9 years), 269 eyes were observed (Sarnicola et al. [38]). This study showed that the ECL was 11% and that this occurred only in the first 6 months after surgery. Later on, no significant ECL was evident, and ECD remained stable afterwards. In a 2-year follow-up study, Shimazaki et al. reported similar results in the DALK group, in contrast to the progressive decrease in the ECD observed in the PK group [70].

Graft Survival

Achieving a better graft survival explains why surgeons choose a surgery with a difficult learning curve.

Postoperative ECD stability is the key reason that made surgeons to move from PK to DALK, not to mention the avoidance of endothelial rejection with host endothelium. However, long-term randomized clinical trials comparing DALK and PK are desirable. Reinhart et al. suggested that these studies are needed even though they are very difficult and onerous to implement. Moreover, randomized prospective comparative studies of DALK and PK might be seen unacceptable by both surgeons and patients, given the advantages provided by DALK in term of ECD and rejection rate: this might represent an unmovable obstacle to enroll patients [36].

Thompson et al. [71] reported the graft survival rate in the largest retrospective case series of PK (3,992 eyes). The survival of the initial grafts was 90% at 5 years and 82% at 10 years. In particular, the highest survival rate was noted in eyes with keratoconus as preoperative diagnosis: 97% at 5 years and 92% at 10 years. The overall survival rate decreased dramatically when regrafting was needed: 53% at 5 years and 41% at 10 years. Graft failure occurred in 10% of the eyes. The most common causes of secondary graft failure were endothelial failure (29%) and immunologic endothelial rejection (27%).

Sarnicola et al. [38] published data about the largest DALK case series (660 eyes) in eyes with different preoperative diagnosis. The mean follow-up duration was 4.5 years (range 0.5–10 years). The average graft survival rate was 99.3% (range 98.5–100%) after up to 10 years of follow-up. The graft failure rate was 0.6%, and occurred only within the first postoperative year, mostly due to ocular surface problems. One year after surgery, ocular surface deficiencies were restored, and ECD was good and stable. This may indicate that after the first postoperative year, DALK graft survival becomes time-independent of and probably lasts lifetime.

Complications

DALK complications can be divided into two broad categories as intraoperative and postoperative.

Intraoperative Complications

Descemet's Membrane Ruptures
DM rupture is the most common complication during DALK surgery, even in experienced hands. Different kinds of ruptures can occur. Microperforation is a small DM lesion that usually occurs during the pdDALK approach when the surgeon tries to go *'deeper and deeper'* with the spatula.

Conversely, macroperforation is a DM rupture that determines an anterior chamber collapse. It generally happens during the removal of residual peripheral stroma using corneal scissors in the dDALK approach.

All DM ruptures were repaired by our study group during the last 12 years (Data under peer review for publication, presented at the VII World Cornea Congress, San Diego 2015, 'DALK: all the ruptures can be fixed'). The ability to repair DM ruptures generally improves when surgeons gradually become more expert. Knowing that DM ruptures can be fixed allows the surgeon to feel more confident in going *deeper and deeper* looking for DM. To our knowledge, the literature does not report detailed explanations regarding the management of DM rupture. For this reason, we are happy to share some personal tips to deal with this complication.

Stromectomy has to be completed to avoid any stromal *'steps'* between the donor and the recipient. Stromal *'steps'* prevent the good and rapid donor-recipient attachment and can keep the DM rupture open.

We would also suggest that the site of the DM break has to be dissected at last stage, after having completed the stromectomy in the remainder descemetic areas. In fact, completing the stromectomy in the DM broken area can enlarge the rupture.

Air can be injected into the anterior chamber only after having sutured the donor. It does not make any sense to inject air into the anterior chamber before having sutured the donor because the surgeon does not obtain any information with this approach and just risks enlarging the rupture.

Finally, it is useful to move the eye in order to remove fluid from the interface. The air bubble has to be left in the anterior chamber for a few hours, positioning the patient's head so that the DM break is sealed (in a semi-sitting position, supine with chin hyperextended using a pillow under the shoulders, etc.). We would recommend a careful monitoring of the patient every two hours in order to drain the air in case of pupillary block, and to prevent a fixed dilated pupil (Urrets-Zavalia syndrome) [72, 73].

Some studies show that DM ruptures and their management cause greater ECL than DALK without DM ruptures [36, 74]. However, it is our conviction that a host endothelium is still better than a donor endothelium, even with greater ECL.

Intraoperative perforation rates vary from 4 to 39% based on five case series, whereas the PK conversion rate has been reported to range from 0 to 14% in four case series [2]. The PK conversion rate gradually decreases as surgeons become more experienced and learn to manage DM ruptures.

The use of fibrin glue for DM break management is controversial [75, 76].

Descemet's Membrane Ruptures in Special Cases: We have already stated that a complete and good stromectomy is needed in cases of DM rupture. By this way, donor tissue can be laid on the recipient bed without any stress.

However, the repair of DM ruptures can be very challenging in some cases. A recipient bed too flat or too steep causes a disparity in curvature between the donor and the recipient, preventing the correct recipient-donor adhesion and leaving the DM ruptures open.

Our study group presented (at the recent VII World Cornea Congress in San Diego, 2015) a suitable technique to repair DM ruptures in these situations by performing a full-thickness total or subtotal circular cut of the recipient bed in order to eliminate any tension and adherence problems.

Full-Thickness Subtotal Circular Cut of the Recipient Bed. This technique is indicated for the management of DM ruptures that happen in pdDALK cases when the recipient bed is significantly *flatter* than the donor graft. In these cases, a full-thickness and subtotal circular cut of the recipient bed, saving a few millimeters of tissue at 6 o'clock, allows for attachment of the recipient bed to the donor graft, after having sutured the donor and injecting an air bubble into the anterior chamber via a limbal paracentesis at 6 o'clock [72] (fig. 15).

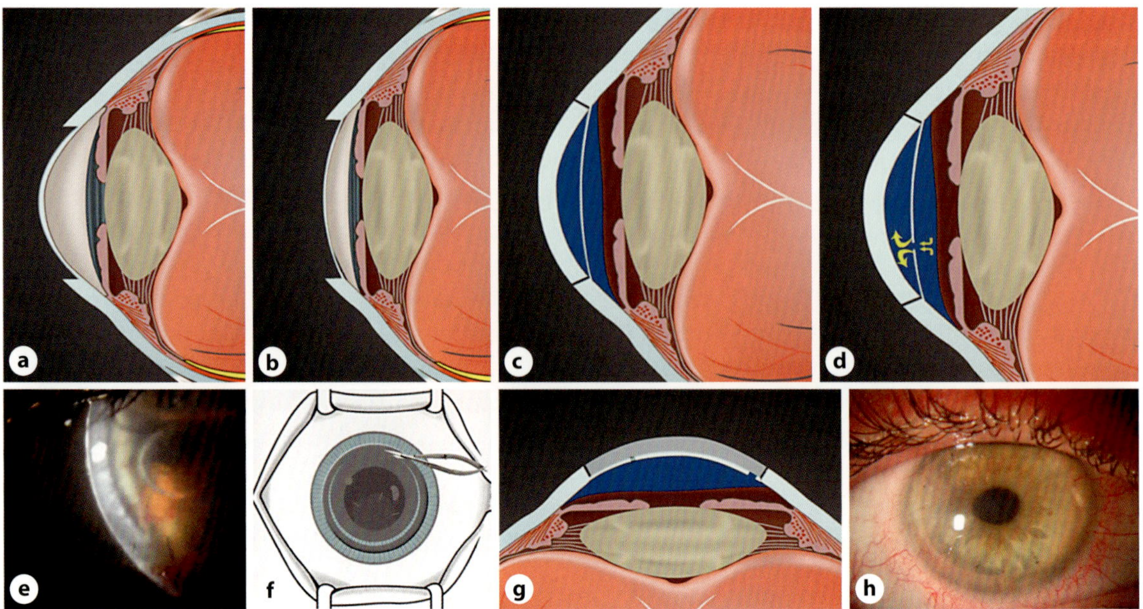

Fig. 15. Full-thickness subtotal circular cut of the recipient bed. **a** Regular DM profile; **b** very flat DM profile; **c–e** a disparity of curvature between the donor graft and the flatter recipient bed causes tension and adherence issues, especially in the presence of DM rupture (yellow arrows); **f** subtotal full-thickness circular bed, leaving an uncut zone of DM at 6 o'clock; **g** DM attached to the donor graft after air bubble injection via paracentesis at 6 o'clock; **h** 1 year postoperative.

Full-Thickness Total Circular Cut of the Recipient Bed. This alternative technique is suitable for the management of DM ruptures that happen in pdDALK cases, in which the recipient bed is significantly *steeper* than the donor graft. In these cases, after stromectomy has been completed, the recipient bed is cut at 360° full-thickness and is attached to the graft button denuded from its endothelium using fibrin glue. The graft made by the donor button and the recipient's endothelium is then sutured, and an air bubble is left in the anterior chamber [72] (fig. 16–18).

Excessive Trephination

Luckily, this is a rare complication that can be avoided by a careful examination of the preoperative pachymetric map and by verifying the trephine calibration. However, if it happens, this complication can be repaired. The BB technique and viscodissection are not indicated. Manual dissection after suturing the perforated area is the most suitable procedure. Layer-by-layer delamination should be performed from the periphery toward the center, without dissecting the perforated area. At this point, the donor graft can be sutured, except in the perforated and undissected area. Stromectomy can then be completed in the perforated area, and finally, the donor graft can be completely sutured. The injection of air into the anterior chamber and the movement of the eye in order to remove interface fluids are the last steps [72] (fig. 19).

Puncturing Descemet's Membrane during the Big Bubble Technique Using a Needle

This is a potential complication observable during the Awar needle-based BB technique. The fear of perforating the DM with the needle makes some surgeons not to go deep enough to reach the BB. This problem has been eliminated with the introduction of the cannula-based BB technique [21].

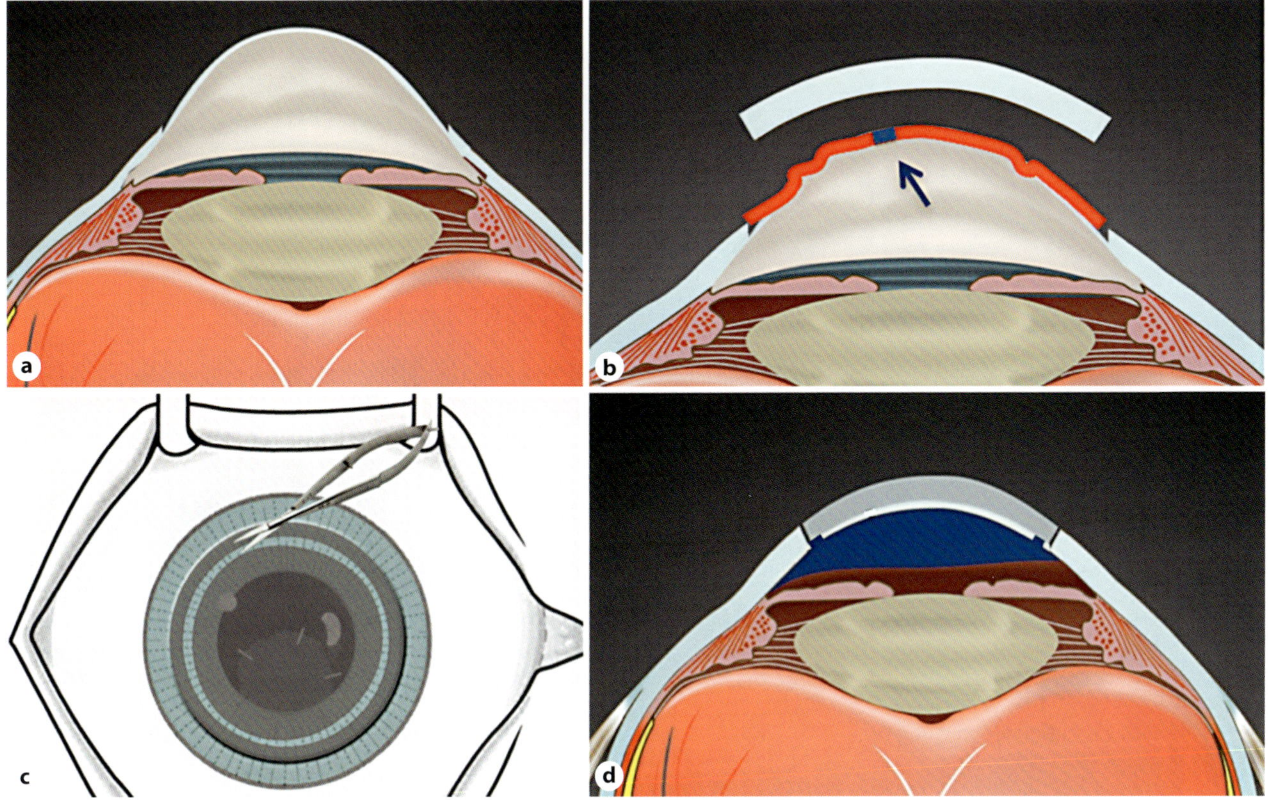

Fig. 16. Full-thickness total circular cut of the recipient bed: scheme. **a** Very steep DM profile in keratoglobus; **b** DM rupture (blue arrow) and disparity of curvature between the donor graft and the steeper recipient bed; **c** Full-thickness 360° circular bed cut of the recipient bed; **d** postoperative: the graft is sutured by gluing the donor stroma to DM of the host.

Descemet's Membrane Disinsertion

DM disinsertion in a quadrant is a rare, even though possible, complication. Our opinion is that it is related to the path found by the air injected into the corneal stroma when it reaches the corneal periphery. In the vast majority of cases, air reaches the anterior chamber through the trabecular meshwork as micro-bubbles. Very rarely, air can cause DM disinsertion in a quadrant of the cornea. In our experience, this has happened in 2 out of more than 1,000 DALK cases [unpublished data]. In both of these cases, the surgery was successfully completed. In one of the two cases, DM was rolled up on itself after 20 days postoperatively (fig. 20), which was probably due to strong eye rubbing by the patient. DM was rolled on itself in the same way it happens during DMEK donor preparation. It required surgical correction performing a redistension of DM and air bubble injection into the anterior chamber [72].

Postoperative Complications

Postoperative complications can be distinguished into early and late complications, depending on whether they occur within or after the first 15 days following surgery.

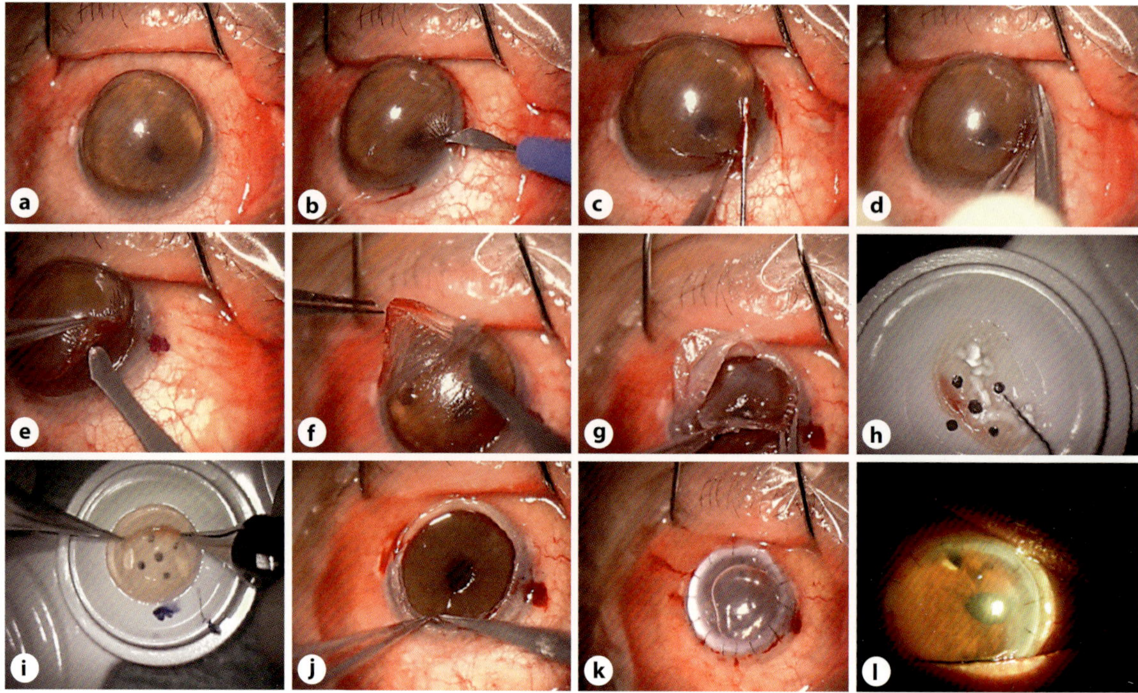

Fig. 17. Full-thickness total circular cut of the recipient bed: surgical steps. **a** Preoperative keratoglobus; **b–e** manual dissection using a smooth spatula, forceps and a Golf knife; **f** DM rupture **g** full-thickness 360° circular cut of the recipient bed; **h, i** the cut recipient bed is preserved and glued to the donor graft lamella, which was previously denuded from its endothelium; **j** completed stromectomy; **k** suturing of the graft made by the donor stroma and DM of the host, followed by air injection into the anterior chamber; **l** postoperative.

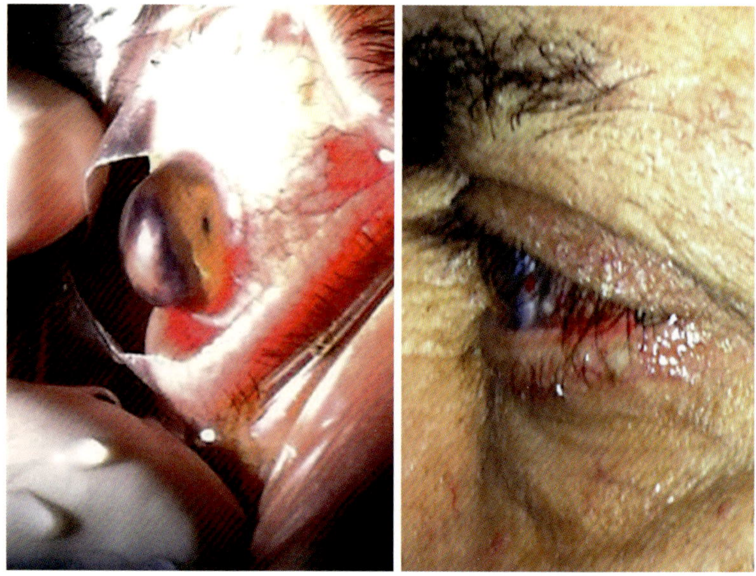

Fig. 18. Keratoglobus: preoperative vs. postoperative.

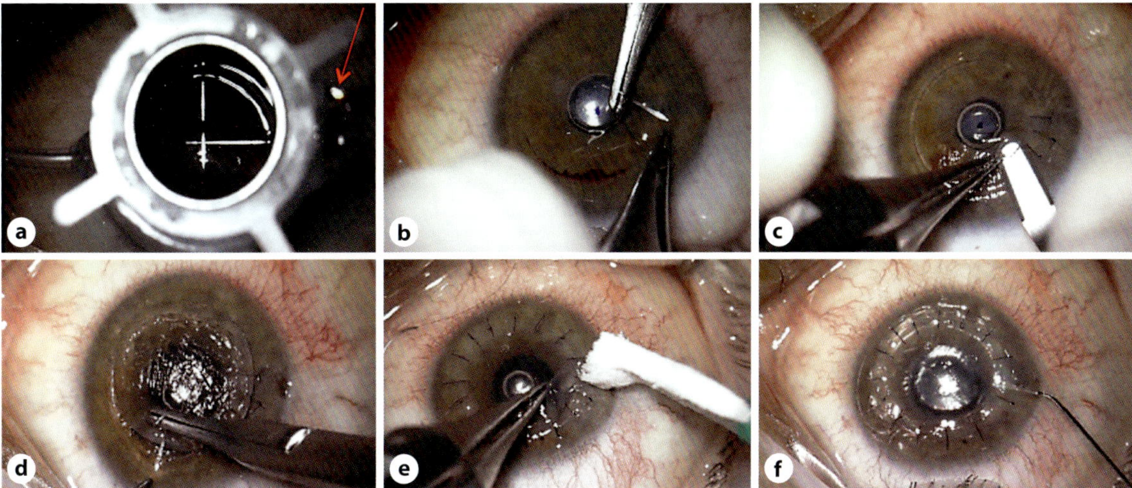

Fig. 19. Excessive trephination. **a** The red arrow shows OVD leakage due to excessive trephination; **b** suturing of the perforated zone; **c** layer-by-layer delamination from the periphery toward the center, performed without dissecting the perforated area; **d** suturing of the donor; **e** zone of perforation delamination; **f** finally, the donor graft is completely sutured, and an air bubble is injected into the anterior chamber.

Early Complications

Rejection. After a DALK procedure, rejection is extremely rare and is easily treatable because it does not involve the endothelium. As reported by various authors, the use of topical steroid prophylaxis in both the early and the late postoperative stages is very heterogeneous.

The rejection rate was reported to be 1% of cases by Reinhart et al. [36], 14% of cases by Feizi et al. (of which 66% had a history of vernal keratoconjunctivitis) [77], and 4% of cases by Sarnicola et al. (none of which were atopic) [38].

Epithelial rejection (1% of cases in the study by Sarnicola et al.) is usually very mild, always reversible with steroid drops, and occurring within the initial postoperative weeks.

Subepithelial rejection and stromal rejection are late complications that will be discussed below.

Double Anterior Chamber. Double anterior chamber is usually, even though not exclusively, a consequence of DM ruptures. Although DM breaks can be fixed, double anterior chamber still happens. To understand the cause of the double chamber, it is useful to consider the different characteristics of the DM ruptures: DM is wavy and loose in dDALK cases and tense in pdDALK cases. The traction exerted by the suture may represent an important factor. We have already described the surgical tips to manage DM ruptures. Air injection into the anterior chamber usually allows its repair, nonetheless if the suture makes a nonuniform compression, it may result in DM detachment at the rupture site, because the ruptures remain open. Once the air in the anterior chamber is reabsorbed, a double chamber occurs. In such cases, it is necessary to resuture the donor graft after having removed the sutures that were too tight. Air has to be left in the anterior chamber at this point to cushion the ruptures, helping the surgeon to verify if the compression by the sutures is homogeneous.

Double anterior chamber has also been described without any intraoperative DM ruptures [78]. In our experience [unpublished data], this has happened in 3 cases out of more than 1,000 DALK procedures. Aside from the possibility that this complication is due to a microperforation that is unrecognized during the surgery, we hypothesize another likely mechanism. We observed a very

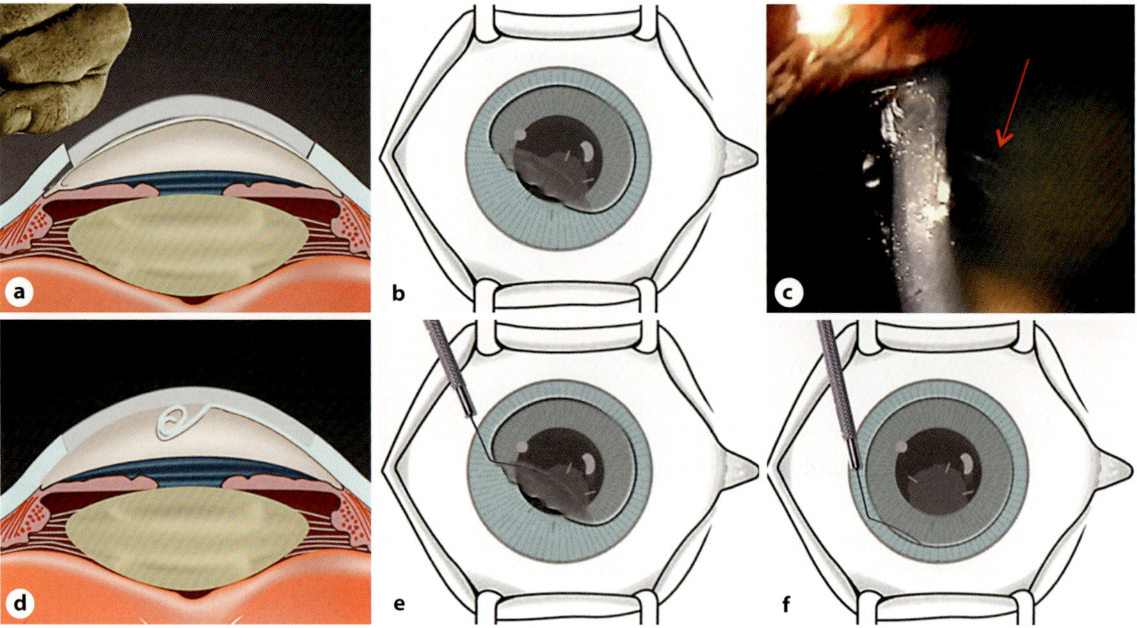

Fig. 20. DM disinsertion. **a** Strong eye rubbing; **b–d** DM rolled-up 20 days postoperatively: scheme and picture (red arrow); **e, f** surgical re-distension of DM and air bubble left in the anterior chamber.

large BB that exceeded the trephination groove in all three of our cases. Considering that our BB technique involves the use of an OVD to facilitate stromal cutting, and to recreate the space between the stroma and DM, once the BB has been opened, we believe that a little bit of viscoelastic material remained in the extreme periphery between DM and the stroma, outside the trephination groove. This material could allow for aqueous percolation from the anterior chamber between DM and the stroma. To manage this complication, we would suggest the injection of air into the anterior chamber, and to perform a 6 o'clock diastasis of the wound between the donor and the recipient at the slit lamp, in order to ensure that the liquid form the interface can flow out autonomously and rapidly.

Descemet's Membrane Wrinkles. DM wrinkles can occur in patients with advanced cones because of disparity of the curvature between the donor and the recipient. Oversizing the donor graft may limit this inconvenience but can also cause a higher spherical equivalent and a more induced myopia. Interrupted suturing can help to manipulate the donor and to displace the DM wrinkles in the periphery, avoiding this negative effect on VA [79]. However, DM wrinkles tend to disappear, or at least to decrease, over time.

Retained Ophthalmic Viscoelastic Device. Retained OVD can happen when the surgeon does not diligently irrigate the host bed before suturing the donor. This can cause a double anterior chamber, making the corneal graft to remain less clear for a long period, until all of the OVD is completely reabsorbed.

Recurrence of the Infection. This complication can occur when DALK surgery is performed for optical purposes in patients with post-herpetic stromal scarring, or as a therapeutic procedure in patients with infectious keratitis unresponsive to medical treatment. The recurrence of herpes simplex virus infection has already been discussed in the 'Indications' section. The risks of infection recurrence following therapeutic DALK are mostly related to the deferral of the intervention. If the infection involves DM, DALK surgery cannot be radical. In order to remove all of the infected corneal tissue, DALK should be performed at the earliest stages of the infection. The pathological examination of the removed lamella is crucial for evaluating the radicality of surgery (Data under peer review for publication, presented at the VII World Cornea Congress, San Diego 2015, 'Precocious DALK in active keratitis poorly responsive to medical treatment').

Interface Haze. This uncommon complication seems to be related to several factors including: keratocyte activation, the depth and the smoothness of the recipient bed, and the healing process at the interface [80]. It usually resolves spontaneously after 4–8 months postoperatively.

In our experience [unpublished data], we noticed that no case of interface haze had occurred since replacing swabs with tying forceps to remove DM from the donor graft. The stromal damage caused by the swabs was probably a cause of keratocyte reactions.

Rare Complications. Rare complications reported in the literature are suture-related complications, dry eye syndrome, microbial infections and transition donor-to-host infections [36].

Late Complications

Subepithelial and Stromal Rejection. Subepithelial rejection is a belated complication that generally happens within the first postoperative year in a range from 3% [38] to 11% of cases [77]; this complication is successfully reversible with topical steroids most of the time. This kind of rejection is usually characterized by decreased vision and nummular infiltrates. It should not be confused with adenovirus keratoconjunctivitis, which has a similar appearance. The differential diagnosis is based on distribution of the infiltrates, which is limited to the donor graft in cases of rejection.

Stromal rejection is a more dangerous complication because it can lead to the necrosis of the stroma. It is usually very rare. Feizi et al. reported this complication at a rate of 3%, reversed in all cases with topical steroids [77]. In our experience (more than 1,000 DALK cases [unpublished data]), stromal rejection has never occurred, probably thanks to a lifetime postoperative therapy with loteprednol eye drops once a day.

Intolerable Astigmatism. Separate removal of the interrupted sutures allows for good management of postoperative astigmatism. Relaxing incisions [81], laser-assisted in situ keratomileusis [82], or Artisan iris-fixed toric phakic intraocular lenses [83] could be good options in selective cases.

Rare Complications. Rare complications reported in the literature include the following: recurrence of corneal stromal dystrophies (especially lattice dystrophy) [40], recurrence of keratoconus [84], epithelial ingrowth [36] and endothelial failure [38].

References

1 Von Hippel A: Eine neue Methode der Hornhaut transplantation. Graefes Arch Ophthal 1888;34:108–130.
2 Tan DT, Dart JK, Holland EJ, et al: Corneal transpantation. Lancet 2012;379:1749–1761.
3 Barraquer JI: Lamellar keratoplasty (special techniques). Ann Ophthalmol 1972;4:437–469.
4 Sarnicola V, Toro P, Gentile D, et al: Descemeti DALK and predescemetic DALK: outcomes in 236 cases of keratoconus. Cornea 2010;29:53–59.
5 Sugita J, Kondo J: Deep lamellar keratoplasty with complete removal of pathological stroma for vision improvement. Br J Ophthalmol 1997;81:184–188.
6 Melles GR, Rietveld FJ, Beekhuis WH, et al: A technique to visualize corneal incision and lamellar dissection depth during surgery. Cornea 1999;18:80–86.
7 Melles GR, Lander F, Rietveld FJ, et al: A new surgical technique for deep stromal, anterior lamellar keratoplasty. Br J Ophthalmol 1999;83:327–333.
8 Anwar M: Dissection technique in lamellar keratoplasty. Br J Ophthalmol 1972;56:711–713.
9 Archila E: Deep lamellar keratoplasty dissection of host tissue with intrastromal air injection. Cornea 1985;3:217–218.
10 Price F: Air lamellar keratoplasty. Refract Corneal Surg 1989;5:240–243.
11 Chau G, Dilly S, Sheard C, et al: Deep lamellar keratoplasty on air with lyophilized tissue. Br J Ophthalmol 1992;76:646–650.

12 Anwar M, Teichmann KD: Big-bubble technique to bare Descemet's membrane in anterior lamellar keratoplasty. J Cataract Refract Surg 2002;28:398–403.

13 Tsubota K, Kaido M, Monden Y, et al: A new surgical technique for deep lamellar keratoplasty with single running suture adjustment. Am J Ophthalmol 1998;126:1–8.

14 Melles GRJ, Remeijer L, Geerards AJM, et al: A quick surgical technique for deep lamellar keratoplasty using visco-dissection. Cornea 2000;19:427.

15 Arenas E, Esquenazi S, Anwar M, et al: Lamellar corneal transpantation. Surv Ophthalmol 2012;57:510–529.

16 Goshe J, Terry MA, Shamie N, et al: Ophthalmic viscosurgical device-assisted incision modification for the big-bubble technique in deep anterior lamellar keratoplasty. J Cataract Refract Surg 2011;37:1923–1927.

17 Parthasarathy A, Por YM, Tan DT: Using a 'small bubble technique' to aid in success in Anwar's 'big bubble technique' of deep lamellar keratoplasty with complete baring of Descemet's membrane. Br J Ophthalmol 2008;92:422.

18 Bausch & Lomb: Fogla DALK instruments, 2009. http://www.storzeye.com/PDF/FoglaDALK_0509_small.pdf.

19 http://www.asico.com/procedures/corneal/corneal-transplant/dalk-deep-anterior-lamellar-keratoplasty/sarnicola-big-bubble-cannula-27g.html#.VVNFTEsd7K8.

20 http://www.asico.com/procedures/corneal/corneal-transplant/dalk-deep-anterior-lamellar-keratoplasty/tan-dalk-cannula-27g.html#.VVNFT0sd7K8.

21 Sarnicola V, Toro P: Blunt cannula for descemetic deep anterior lamellar keratoplasty. Cornea 2011;30:895–898.

22 Fournié P, Malecaze F, Coullet J, et al: Variant of the big bubble technique in deep anterioir lamellar keratoplasty. J Cataract Refract Surg 2007;33:371–375.

23 Muftuoglu O, Toro P, Hogan RN, et al: Sarnicola air-visco bubble technique in deep anterior lamellar keratoplasty. Cornea 2013;32:527–532.

24 Shimmura S, Ando M, Ishioka M, et al: Same-size donor corneas for myopic keratoconus. Cornea 2004;23:345–349.

25 Chan CC, Ritenour RJ, Kumar NL, et al: Femtosecond laser assisted mushroom configuration deep anterior lamellar keratoplasty. Cornea 2010;29:290–295.

26 Farid M, Steinert RF: Deep anterior lamellar keratoplasty performed with the femtosecond laser zigzag incision for the treatment os stromal corneal pathology and ectatic diseases. J Cataract Refract Surg 2009;35:809–813.

27 Price FW Jr, Price MO, Grading JC, et al: Deep anterior lamellar keratoplasty with femtosecond-laser zigzag incisions. J Cataract Refract Surg 2009;35:804–808.

28 Buzzonetti L, Petrocelli G, Valente P: Femtosecond laser and big-bubble deep anterior lamellar keratoplasty: a new chance. J Ophthalmol 2012;2012:264590.

29 Shehadeh-Mashor R, Chan C, Yeung SN, et al: Long-term outcomes of femtosecond laser-assisted mushroom configuration deep anterior lamellar keratoplasty. Cornea 2013;32:390–395.

30 Shehadeh-Mashor R, Chan CC, Bahar I, et al: Comparison between femtosecond laser mushroom configuration and manual trephine straight-edge configuration deep anterior lamellar keratoplasty. Br J Ophthalmol 2014;98:35–39.

31 Ghanem RC, Ghanem MA: Pachymetry-guided itrastromal air injection ('pachy-bubble') for deep anterior lamellar keratoplasty. Cornea 2012;31:1087–1091.

32 Riss S, Heindl LM, Bachmann BO, et al: Pentacam-based big bubble deep anterior lamellar keratoplasty in patients with keratoconus. Cornea 2012;31:627–632.

33 Scorcia V, Busin M, Lucisano A, et al: Anterior segment optical coherence tomography-guided big-bubble technique. Ophthalomolgy 2013;120:471–476.

34 De Benito-Llopis L, Metha JS, Angunawela RI, et al: Intraoperative anterior segment optical coherence tomography: a novel assessment tool during deep anterior lamellar keratoplasty. Am J Ophthalmol 2014;157:334–341.e3.

35 Luengo-Gimeno F, Tan DT, Metha JS: Evolution of deep anterior lamellar keratoplasty (DALK). Ocul Surf 2011;9:98–110.

36 Reinhart WJ, et al: Deep anterior lamellar keratoplasty as an alternative to penetrating keratoplasty a report by the American Academy of Ophthalmology. Ophtalmology 2011;118:209–218.

37 Karimian F, Feizi S: Deep anterior lamellar keratoplasty: indications, surgical techniques and complications. Middle East Afr J Ophthalmol 2010;17:28–37.

38 Sarnicola V, Toro P, Sarnicola C, et al: Long-term graft survivall in deep anterior lamellar keratoplasty. Cornea 2012;31:621–626.

39 Fogla R: Deep anterior lamellar keratoplasty in the management of keratoconus. Indian J Ophthalmol 2013;61:465–468.

40 Unal M, Arslan OS, Atalay E, et al: Deep anterior lamellar keratoplasty for the treatment of stromal corneal dystrophies. Cornea 2013;32:301–305.

41 Cheng J, Qi X, Zhao J, et al: Comparison of penetrating keratoplasty and deep lamellar keratoplasty for macular corneal dystrophy and risk factors of recurrence. Opthalmology 2013;120:34–39.

42 Sogutulu Sari E, Kubaloglu A, Unal M, et al: Deep anterior lamellar keratoplasty versus penetrating keratoplasty for macular corneal dystrophy: a randomized trial. Am L Ophthalmol 2013;156:267–274.

43 Park KA, Ki CS, Chung ES, et al: Deep anterior lamellar keratoplasty in Korean patients with Avellino dystrophy. Cornea 2007;26:1132–1135.

44 Vajpayee RB, Tyagi J, Sharma N, et al: Deep anterior lamellar keratoplasty by big-bubble technique for treatment corneal stromal opacities. Am J Opthalmol 2007;143:954–957.

45 Harding SA, Nischal KK, Upponi-Patil A, et al: Indications and outcomes of deep anterior amellar keratoplasty in children. Ophthalmology 2010;17:2191–2195.

46 Millar MJ, Maloof A: Deep lamellar keratoplasty for pellucid marginal degeneration: review of management options for corneal perforation. Cornea 2008;27:953–956.

47 Anshu A, Paratharsarathy A, Metha JS, et al: Outcomes of therapeutic deep lamellar keratoplasty for advanced infectious keratitis: a comparative study. Ophthalmology 2009;116:615–623.

48 Parathasarathy A, Tan DT: Deep lamellar keratoplasty for acanthamoeba keratitis. Cornea 2007;26:1021–1023.

49 Ang M, Metha JS, Manthoo S, et al: Deep anterior lamellar keratoplasty to treat microsporidial stromal keratitis. Cornea 2009;28:832–835.

50 Sarnicola V, Toro P: Deep anterior lamellar keratoplasty in herpes simplex corneal opacities. Cornea 2010;29:60–64.

51 Wu SQ, Zhou P, Zhang B, et al: Long-term comparison of full-bed deep lamellar keratoplasty with penetrating keratoplasty in treating corneal leucoma caused by herpes simplex keratitis. Am J Ophthalmol 2012;153:291–299.

52 Leccisotti A: Air-assisted manual deep anterior lamellar keratoplasty for treatment of herpetic corneal scars. Cornea 2009;28:728–731.

53 Awan MA, Roberts F, Hegarty B, et al: The outcome of deep anterior lamellar keratoplasty in herpes simplex virus-related corneal scarring, complications and graft survival. Br J Ophthalmol 2010;94:1300–1303.

54 Wang J, Zhao G, Xie L, et al: Therapeutic effect of deep anterior lamellar keratoplasty for active or quiescent herpetic stromal keratitis. Graefes Arch Clin Exp Ophthalmol 2012;250:1187–1194.

55 Chiou AG, Bovet J, de Courten C: Management of Corenal ectasia and cataract following photorefractive keratectomy. J Cataract Refract Surg 2006;32:679–680.

56 McAllum PJ, Segev F, Herzig S, et al: Deep anterior lamellar keratoplasty for post-LASIK ectasia. Cornea 2007;26:507–511.

57 Villarubia A, Pérez-Santonja JJ, Palacín E, et al: Deep anterior lamellar keratoplasty in post-laser in situ keratomileusis keratectasia. J Cataract Refract Surg 2007;33:773–778.

58 Ramamurthi S, Cornish KS, Steeples L, et al: Deep anterior lamellar keratoplasty on a previously failed full-thickness graft. Cornea 2009;28:456–457.

59 Lake D, Hamada S, Khan S, et al: Deep anterior lamellar keratoplasty over penetrating keratoplasty for host rim thinning and ectasia. Cornea 2009;28:489–492.

60 Singh G, Singh Bhinder H: Evaluation of therapeutic deep anterior lamellar keratoplastyin acute ocular chemical burns. Eur J Ophthalmol 2008;18:517–528.

61 Fogla R, Padmanabhan P: Deep anterior lamellar keratoplasty combined with autologous limbal stem cell transplantation in unilateral severe chemical injury. Cornea 2005;24:421–425.

62 Sharma N, Kumar C, Mannan R, et al: Surgical technique of deep anterior lamellar keratoplasty in descemetoceles. Cornea 2010;29:1448–1451.

63 Gabison EE, Doan S, Catanese M, et al: Modified deep anterior lamellar keratoplasty in the management of small and large descemetoceles. Cornea 2011;30:1179–1182.

64 Shimmura S, Shimazaki J, Tsubota K: Therapeutic deep lamellar keratoplasty for cornea perforation. Am J Ophthalmol 2003;135:896–897.

65 Bhatt PR, Lim LT, Ramaesh K: Therapeutic deep lamellar keratoplasty for corneal perforations. Eye (Lond) 2007;21:1168–1173.

66 Han DC, Metha JS, Por YM, et al: Comparison ofoutcomes of lamellar keratoplasy and penetrating keratoplasty in keratoconus. Am L Ophthalmol 2009;148:744–751.

67 Bhatt UK, Fares U, Rahman I, et al: Outcomes of deep anterior lamellar keratoplasty following successful and failed 'big bubble'. Br J Ophthalmol 2012;96:564–569.

68 Fontana L, Parente G, Sincich A, et al: Influence of graft-host interface on the quality of vision after deep anterior lamellar keratoplasty in patients with keratoconus. Cornea 2011;30:497–502.

69 Ardjomand N, Hau S, McAlister JC, et al: Quality of vision and graft thickness in deep anterior lamellar and penetrating corneal allografts. Am J Ophthalmol 2007;143:228–235.

70 Shimazaki J, Shimmura S, Ishioka M, et al: Randomized clinical trial of deep lamellar keratoplasty vs penetrating keratoplasty. Am J Ophthalmol 202;134:159–165.

71 Thompson RW Jr, Price MO, Bowers PJ, et al: Long-term graft survival after penetrating keratoplasty. Ophthalmology 2003;110:1396–1402.

72 Cornea fourth edition. Mark J. Mannis and Edward J. Holland Part IX: Keratoplasty. Section 4: Lamellar keratoplasty. Chapter 120 'Recovery techniques in DALK'. Elsevier, in press.

73 Maurino V, Allan BD, Stevens JD, et al: Fixed dilated pupil (Urrets-Zavalia syndrome) afetr air7gas injection after deep anterior lamellar keratoplasty for keratoconus. Am J Ophthalmol 2002;133:266–268.

74 Leccisotti A: Descemet's membrane perforation during deep anterior lamellar keratoplasty: prognosis. J Cataract Refract Surg 2007;33:825–829.

75 Por YM, Tan YL, Metha JS, et al: Intracameral fibrin tissue sealant as an adjunct in tectonic lamellar keratoplasty for large perforations. Cornea 2009;28:451–455.

76 Anwar HM, El-Danasoury A, Hashem AN: The use of fibrin glue to seal Descemet membrane microperforations occurring during deep anterior lamellar keratoplasty. Cornea 2012;31:1193–1196.

77 Feizi S, Javadi MA, Jamali H, et al: Deep anterior lamellar keratoplasty in patients with keratoconus: big-bubble technique. Cornea 2010;29:177–182.

78 Mohamed-Noriega K, Metha JS: Sweating of Descemet's membrane during deep anterior lamellar kearoplasty in absence of perforation. Clin Ophthalmol 2012;6:1441–1443.

79 Shi W, Li S, Gao H, et al: Modified deep lamellar keratoplasty for the treatment of advanced-stage keratoconus with steep curvature. Ophthalmology 2010;117:226–231.

80 Abdelkader A, Kaufan HE: Descemetic versus pre-descemetic lamellar keratoplasty: clinical and confocal study. Cornea 2011;30:1244–1252.

81 Javadi MA, Feizi S, Mirababaee F, et al: Relaxing incisions combined with adjustment sutures for post-deep anterior lamellar keratoplasty astigmatism in keratoconus. Cornea 2009;28:1130–1134.

82 Acar BT, Utine CA, Acar S, et al: Laser in situ keratomileusis to manage refractive errors after deep antertior lamellar keratoplasty. J Cataract Refract Surg 2012;38:1020–1027.

83 Al-Dreihi MG, Louka BI, Anbari AA: Artisan iris-fixated toric phakic intraocular lens for the correction of high astigmatism after deep anterior lamellar keratoplasty. Digit J Ophthalmol 2013;19:39–41.

84 Feizi S, Javadi MA, Rezaei Kanavi M: Recurrent keratoconus in corneal graft after deep anterior lamellar keratoplasty. J Ophthalmic Vis Res 2012;7:328–331.

Enrica Sarnicola, MD
University of Siena
Via Mazzini n°62
IT–58100 Grosseto (Italy)
E-Mail e.sarnicola@hotmail.it

Güell JL (ed): Cornea. ESASO Course Series. Basel, Karger, 2015, vol 6, pp 102–123
DOI: 10.1159/000381496

Descemet Membrane Endothelial Keratoplasty: Update on Endothelial Transplantation Techniques

Jose L. Güell[a, b] · Mohamed El Husseiny[d] · Merce Morral[c] · Oscar Gris[a] · Manero Felicidad[a]

[a] IMO. Instituto Microcirugia Ocular (IMO) of Barcelona and [b] Auitonoma University of Barcelona and [c] Department of Cornea and Anterior Segment Disease and Refractive Surgery, Institut Clinic d'Oftalmologia, Hospital Clinic i Provincial, Barcelona, Spain; [d] Research Institute of Ophthalmology (RIO), Giza, Egypt

Abstract

The cornea remains in a state of deturgescence, maintained by the endothelial cell Na+/K+ ATPase and by tight junctions between endothelial cells that limit the entrance of fluid into the stroma. By maintaining an optimum level of corneal hydration, endothelial cells preserve the ordered arrangement of collagen fibers, which is crucial for corneal transparency. Fuchs' endothelial corneal dystrophy (FECD) was initially described by Fuchs in 1910 as a combination of epithelial and stromal edema in older patients. It manifests itself as bilateral, albeit asymmetric, central corneal guttae, corneal edema, and reduced vision. The Descemet membrane thickens and develops excrescences known histopathologically as guttae. Stromal edema develops, and the corneal thickness may increase to over 1,000 μm. When the edema is severe, the corneal epithelium can detach from its basement membrane, creating painful bullae on the anterior surface of the cornea. FECD is the most common endothelial dystrophy and is usually seen beyond the fifth decade of life, although not all cases are in the elderly. Pseudophakic bullous keratopathy is a term used to describe endothelial cell loss caused by surgical manipulations in the anterior chamber (usually due to pseudophakic intraocular lens (IOL) implantation, but it may be related to any other intraocular surgical procedure, obviously including phakic IOL implantation). If the corneal endothelium is damaged during surgery (as often occurs during cataract extraction, phakic IOL implantation and other procedures), the same spectrum of symptoms as found in FECD can develop, although the histological phenotype of both diseases is different and, usually, there is no guttata in pseudophakic bullous keratopathy. Full-thickness grafts have been the standard of care for treating medically uncontrollable endothelial disease for a significant number of years worldwide. However, although the success rate is 90% in low-risk patients, it is only 30–50% in more complex, higher-risk cases, and overall, 30% of cases have a rejection episode. Moreover, regrafting has become the most common indication for corneal transplantation in the US and in some places in Europe. The more recently developed lamellar keratoplasty techniques are designed to overcome some of the problems of corneal transplantation by leaving as much of the healthy cornea in place as possible. For example, endothelial keratoplasty procedures replace only the endothelium but leave the patient's cornea's refraction as well as most of its biomechanical properties fairly intact. In this chapter, we will review the actual techniques for endothelial transplantation and provide an update on the surgical strategy (mostly for Descemet membrane endothelial keratoplasty) and its clinical results and complications.

Introduction

The adult human cornea averages 540 µm in thickness [1], with the following classical layers, from anterior to posterior: epithelium, epithelial basement membrane, Bowman's layer, stroma, Descemet membrane (DM), and endothelium (fig. 1).

The cornea remains in a state of deturgescence, maintained by the endothelial cell Na+/K+ ATPase and by tight junctions between endothelial cells that limit the entrance of fluid into the stroma. By maintaining an optimum level of corneal hydration, endothelial cells preserve the ordered arrangement of collagen fibers, which is crucial for corneal transparency [2]. When the endothelial cell density is low or the cells are malfunctioning, the associated loss of tight junctions between cells allows more fluid to enter the stroma. The endothelial cells that remain may present a higher concentration of the Na+/K+ ATPase in an effort to compensate for the loss [1].

The average human cornea has an endothelial cell density of 5,000–6,000 cells/mm^2 at birth, decreasing to 2,500–3,000 cells/mm^2 by adulthood. There is an average physiological cell loss of 0.6% per year [1]. Corneal edema appears at 700–400 cells/mm^2 [1, 3]. Adult human corneal endothelial cells are arrested in the G phase of the cell cycle and do not undergo mitosis [4]. Therefore, lost cells cannot be replaced physiologically, although, as we will see throughout this chapter, significant research is focused on this subject.

Fuchs' endothelial corneal dystrophy (FECD) was initially described by Fuchs in 1910 as a combination of epithelial and stromal edema in older patients [5]. It manifests itself as bilateral, albeit asymmetric, central corneal guttae, corneal edema, and reduced vision [6, 7]. The DM thickens

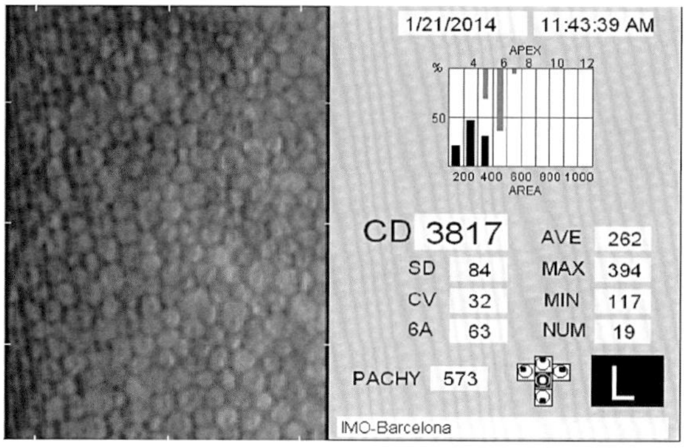

Fig. 1. Microscopy view of a young healthy endothelium.

and develops excrescences known histopathologically as guttae. Stromal edema develops, and the corneal thickness may increase to over 1,000 µm. When the edema is severe, the corneal epithelium can detach from its basement membrane, creating painful bullae on the anterior surface of the cornea [2, 8]. FECD is the most common endothelial dystrophy (the others have the same indications for surgery but, from the perspective of statistical incidence, are almost insignificant) and is usually seen beyond the fifth decade of life, although not all cases are in the elderly; Biswas et al. reported several families with early onset of this dystrophy in the third and fourth decades of life [9]. FECD is, despite its dominant inheritance form, more common and progressive in women [10]. It may also present in a sporadic form and is thought to be a primary disorder of the endothelium, although other hypotheses have been postulated, including some secondary options. The total number of endothelial cells is low, and existing cells may not function properly. The course of this dystrophy can be further accelerated after intraocular surgery, and most commonly cataract extraction. A cell count of less than 1,000 cells/mm^2 and a corneal thickness greater than 640 µm have been classically considered major risk factors for corneal decompensation after cataract surgery [11–13].

Pseudophakic bullous keratopathy (PBK) is a term used to describe endothelial cell loss caused

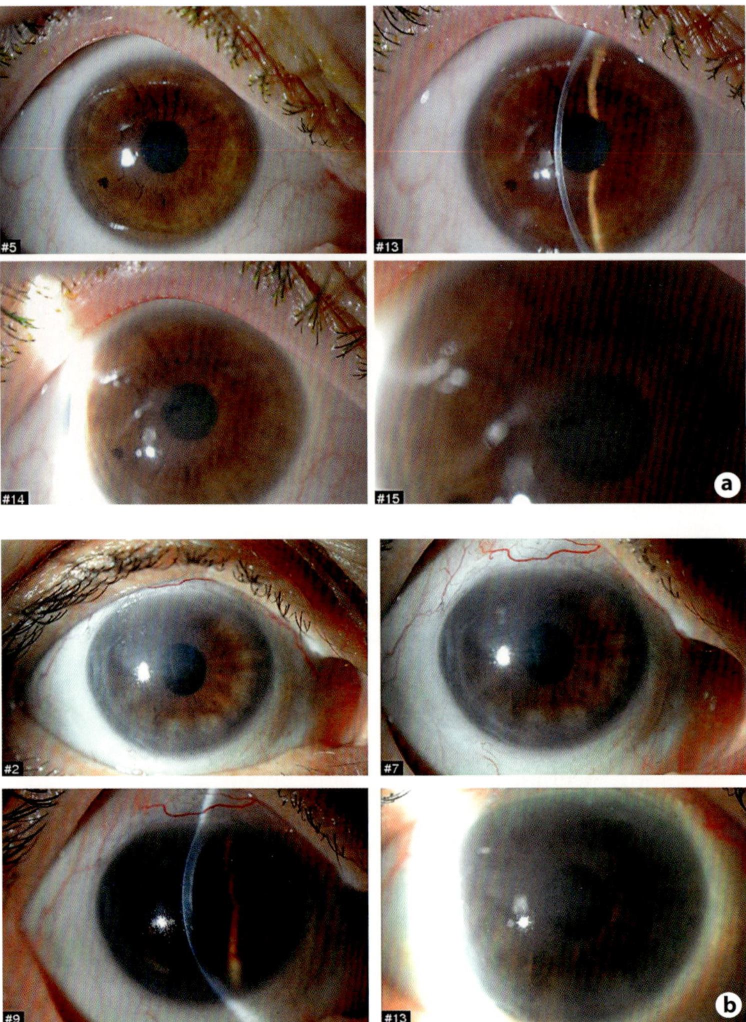

Fig. 2. a Slit-lamp images of an eye with stromal corneal edema and Fuchs' dystrophy and **b** an eye with pseudophakic non-Fuchs' irreversible corneal edema postoperatively.

by surgical manipulations in the anterior chamber (AC). If the corneal endothelium is damaged during surgery (as often occurs during cataract extraction, phakic intraocular lens implantation and other procedures) [3], the same spectrum of symptoms as found in FECD can develop, although the histological phenotype of both diseases is different and, usually, there is no guttata in PBK (fig. 2).

Toxic anterior segment syndrome is a rare complication of intraocular surgery that has only recently been recognized [14]. It is characterized by acute sterile inflammation in the anterior segment caused by noxious agents such as medications, residual viscoelastic agents, or preservatives or by an altered osmolarity or pH of the irrigating solution [15–17]. Permanent corneal endothelial damage can occur in severe cases of toxic anterior segment syndrome.

Full-thickness grafts (PK) have been the standard of care for treating medically uncontrollable endothelial disease for a significant number of years worldwide. Lamellar keratoplasty (LKP) techniques are continuing to gain wider acceptance, although there will likely remain a place for

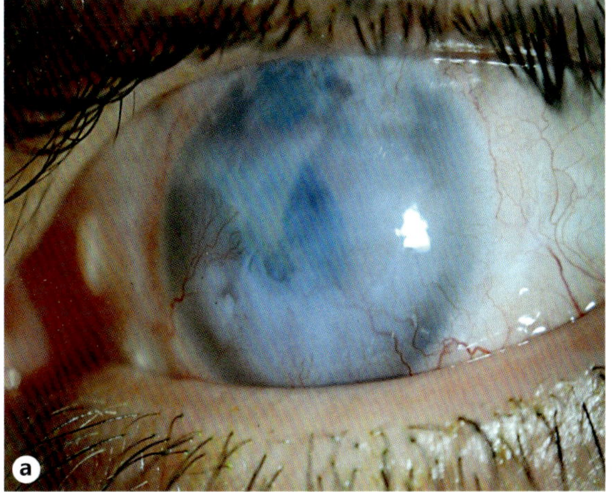

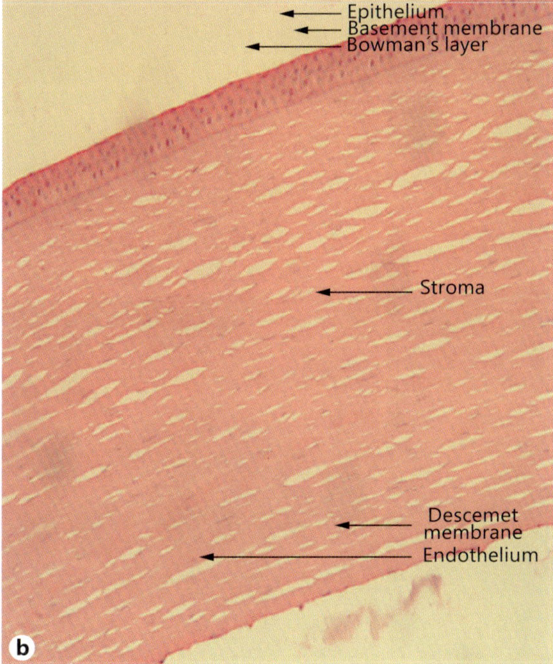

Fig. 3. a Completely opacified corneal candidate for penetrating surgery. **b** Main layers of the human cornea.

30% of cases have a rejection episode. Moreover, regrafting has become the most common indication for corneal transplantation in the US and in some places in Europe.

The more recently developed LKP techniques are designed to overcome some of the problems of corneal transplantation by leaving as much of the healthy cornea in place as possible. For example, endothelial keratoplasty (EK) procedures replace only the endothelium but leave the patient's cornea's refraction fairly intact. In contrast, anterior LKP replaces all or nearly all of the entire cornea, except the DM and the endothelium, which all but grossly eliminates the chance of immune rejection.

In any case, there will always be some FECD and PBK cases in which EK may not be the best option, including eyes in which the anterior stroma is seriously compromised and some circumstances in which eyes are likely to need multiple intraocular procedures, such as anterior vitrectomy, iris reconstruction, or tube implantation (fig. 3a, b).

History of Endothelial Keratoplasty

The history of EK began in 1956, when Tillet published the first description of posterior LKP [18]. Although he used a full-thickness, large incision, it was the first attempt to use the inner layer of the cornea to treat corneal diseases of the endothelium. In the 1960s, Dr. Jose Ignacio Barraquer described a method of EK using an anterior approach via laser-assisted in situ keratomileusis flap formation [19]. After cutting a partial-thickness flap with a microkeratome, the posterior cornea, consisting of stroma, the DM, and endothelium was trephined and replaced with a donor graft that was sutured into place. The flap was then replaced and also sutured. This approach was later employed by different investigators, with variable good results [20], and our personal experience was anatomically very good but yielded poor visual results [21] (fig. 4a–l).

penetrating keratoplasty (PKP) for the foreseeable future. Corneal transplants are the most common solid organ transplants performed around the world. However, although the success rate is 90% in low-risk patients, it is only 30–50% in more complex, higher-risk cases, and overall,

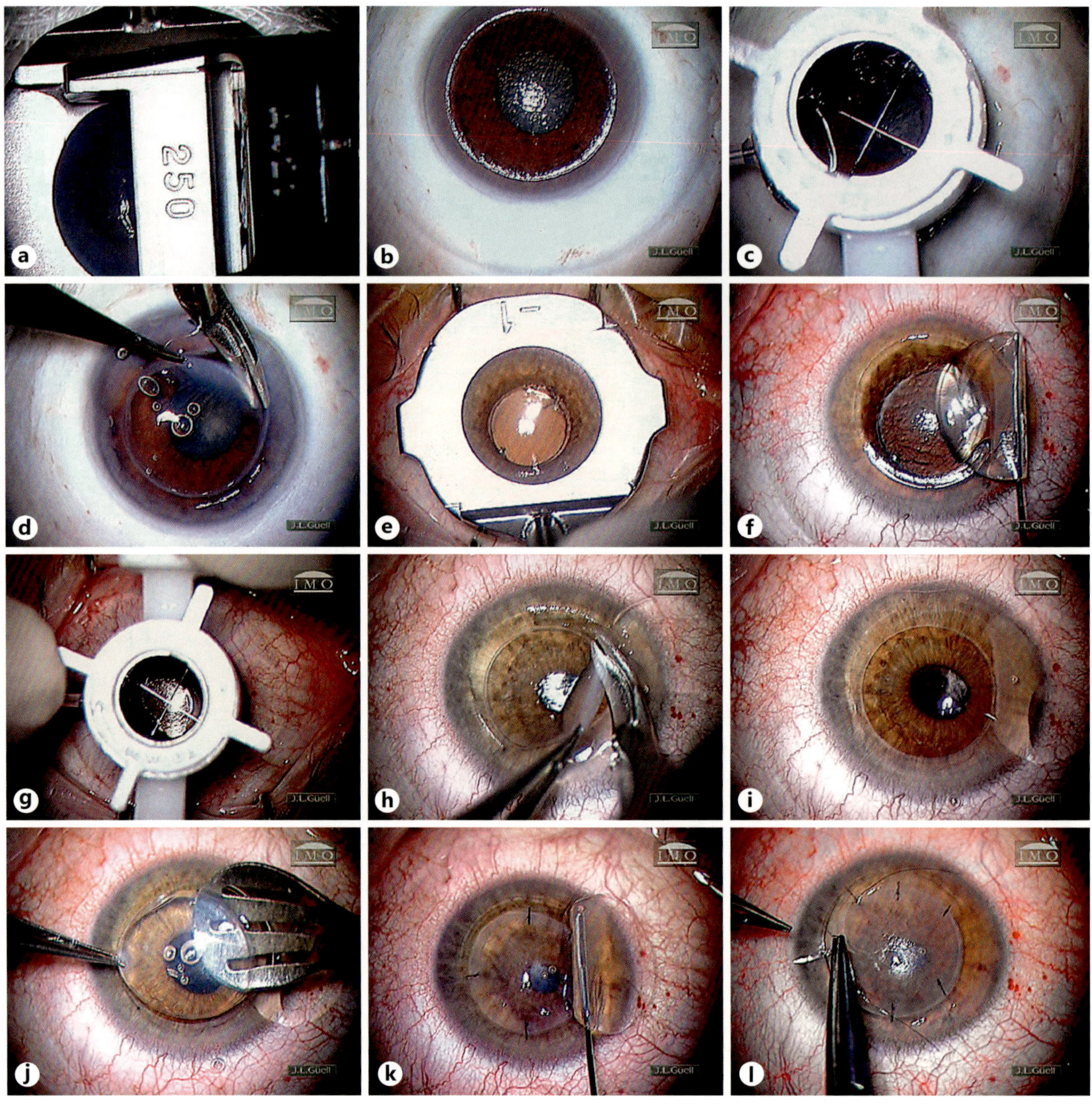

Fig. 4. This is a series of surgical photographs demonstrating the technique originally described many years ago. Using a donor globe and after a microkeratome pass, we obtained an 8-mm specimen with a Hessburg-Barron trephine (posterior 100 µm of stroma, Descemet membrane (DM) and endothelium). On the recipient side, we first created a thick flap and afterward created a trephination of 8 mm in diameter. The donor lenticule was secured by means of 2 or 3 10.0 nylon sutures, and the flap was also sutured with 4 or 5 interrupted 10.0 nylon sutures.

In 1999, Melles et al. directed the field toward an intrastromal approach, describing large-pocket dissection through a sclero-corneal pocket incision that held a donor cornea without sutures [22, 23]. Their technique of posterior LKP avoided some of the pitfalls of full-thickness surgery but involved difficult dissection of both the donor and the host. One of the major advantages, however, was the use of air instead of sutures to initially secure the donor tissue. Sutures that add an anterior

Güell · El Husseiny · Morral · Gris · Felicidad

surgical approach have been associated with a number of complications, including, but not limited to, breakage; infections; and, of course, those risks associated with PK, such as acute glaucoma, rejection and higher fragility when confronted by blunt ocular trauma. At the same time, the point sources of tension from sutures and the alignment of full-thickness stromal cuts are major contributors to the unpredictable variations in both regular and irregular astigmatism postoperatively [24].

Later on, Melles et al. started to change host dissection using simple 'descemetorhexis' in a procedure known as 'Descemet's stripping EK' (DSEK) [25]. Their internal approach of removing the DM from the host left an ultrasmooth posterior surface on which the dissected donor stromal disc could be easily fixed.

Gorovoy proposed the use of a microkeratome to harvest the donor tissue to perform Descemet's stripping automated EK (DSAEK) [26].

At the same time, other modifications, such as the use of local anesthesia, a reverse Sinskey hook, surface compression, and 'venting' corneal incisions, adopted by a high volume very good corneal surgeons, such as Price and Terry in the US, made this procedure the actual standard of care worldwide (for example, the number and percentage of grafts performed via EK increased from 1,429 (3%) in 2005 to approximately 14,159 (28%) in 2007 in the US) [27].

Following the widespread adoption of DSAEK surgery, the Melles group revisited selective DM transplantation and reported the results of a new procedure, or DMEK (DMEK) [28]. In DMEK, the donor DM was stripped from the corneoscleral rim and injected into the host anterior segment, which had been stripped of its own DM, via a 3-mm clear corneal incision. The membrane was unrolled using pneumatic and fluidic manipulations and opposed to the recipient posterior stroma using the air bubble technique. The initial results were encouraging: of 10 eyes transplanted, four had a best-corrected visual acuity (BCVA) better than 20/40 1 week after surgery, and six achieved greater than 20/40 BCVA at week 6 postoperatively. Moreover, this simplified technique negated the need for an automated microkeratome to smooth a stromal graft conceptually, allowing this technique to be accessible to a greater number of surgeons, despite its higher technical difficulty. The Melles group subsequently presented their first 50 cases of DMEK; of those eyes in which the DM graft adhered (n = 40, 80%), 75% achieved a best spectacle-corrected visual acuity of 20/25 or better within 3 months [29].

In December 2009, 2 months after the Melles paper was published, Price et al. reported their prospective study of 60 DMEK procedures in 56 eyes in the US. Their results were similar to those of the Melles study; the Price group reported that 63% of eyes had a BCVA of 20/25 or better initially and that 94% had vision of 20/40 or better at 3 months [30]. This was significantly better than the results achieved with DSAEK surgery.

Initial endothelial cell counts following DMEK were comparable with those following PK or DSAEK. The Melles group reported an average endothelial cell density of 1,850 cells/mm^2 at 6 months after surgery and 1,680 cells/mm^2 at 12 months [31]. The Price group reported a mean endothelial cell loss of 30% at 3 months [30]. These results are similar to values reported after DSEK, DSAEK and PK [32–36].

What Are the Indications and Contraindications for Endothelial Keratoplasty?

EK is the treatment of choice for any patient with endothelial dysfunction that has become visually disabling because EK is safer and provides faster visual recovery than the alternative, or full-thickness PKP [37–39]. Candidates for EK include patients with any type of endothelial dysfunction, including endothelial dystrophies, such as FECD or posterior polymorphous dystrophy; pseudophakic or aphakic bullous keratopathy; iridocorneal endothelial syndrome; endothelial decompensation due to trauma caused by glaucoma tubes; or a failed penetrating graft [37–43].

In eyes with stromal opacity or scarring that would limit postoperative visual potential after EK, replacement of the full corneal thickness with PK is a better choice. In addition, we have found that eyes with even borderline hypotony should not be treated with EK because the graft generally does not clear well in such cases.

Patients particularly appreciate the rapid visual recovery and minimal restrictions on their postoperative physical activity with EK [38, 39]. In fact, since EK is performed with a small incision, essentially no activity restrictions are necessary after 2 months, and patients can even engage in regular contact sports that carry some risk of minor trauma to the eye, such as basketball. This is a significant improvement over standard PK, after which minor trauma can readily rupture the transplant incision and cause loss of the eye [44].

Furthermore, corneal sensation is retained with EK, which helps to minimize or eliminate ocular surface complications.

The improved risk-to-benefit ratio for patients undergoing EK has lowered the threshold when determining who is an appropriate candidate for the procedure. When PK were the only surgical option, patients would often postpone transplantation as long as possible, typically until well after they had seriously curtailed normal daily activities, such as reading and driving. EK provides relatively rapid and predictable visual recovery, so that many patients choose to have EK before their visual disabilities become severe. It is not uncommon for patients with Fuchs' dystrophy to ask for EK when their cornea guttata begins to cause uncomfortable glare while driving or reading under fluorescent lights, even while Snellen acuity in a darkened room is still in the 20/40 range. Visual recovery is so rapid after EK that many patients want to have their second eye treated within a few months of the first eye.

Early treatment of endothelial dysfunction generally produces the most rapid corneal clearing and visual recovery, and some eyes can achieve 20/20 vision within a week of EK. Visual recovery typically takes longer in eyes with long-standing corneal edema or bullous changes. In these eyes, the corneal thickness usually decreases rapidly after EK, but the stroma may retain a whitish or granular appearance for several months up to 2 years. Stromal remodeling by keratocytes appears to progress from the periphery inward, with the central area over the pupil clearing last. Despite the slower visual recovery in eyes with long-standing edema, EK is still the procedure of choice for these patients because it is safer than PK. PK can also entail a prolonged recovery period, with the added burdens of suture-related issues and the potential for irregular astigmatism.

Although we generally prefer to perform cataract surgery before transplantation, in a separate surgical procedure, there are no contraindications for doing it at the same time or for doing it in phakic eyes. It can also be indicated for failed penetrating grafts; for the presence of glaucoma tubes or intraocular lenses in the AC in cases with a shallow AC; or, with more technical difficulties, in those eyes with iris abnormalities, aniridia and/or aphakia [45–47].

Donor Preparation

Preparation of the donor cornea for EK may be performed by the surgeon immediately before the surgery or by the eye bank just before tissue shipment, which is referred to as 'pre-cut tissue'. To minimize endothelial damage, excessive manipulation of the donor as well as a prolonged storage time in Optisol GS should be avoided. In some of the most recent studies, it looks like we can safely store split tissue for up to 1 week in organ culture [48].

Different methods and techniques that are obviously related to the EK technique that the surgeon will use and his own preferences have been described: manual dissection, automated microkeratome dissection, and femtosecond laser dissection as the main options for DSEK and DSAEK and more specific techniques for DMEK, such as the SCUBA (submerged cornea using backgrounds away) technique [49–55].

At the same time, we are still evaluating the best technique for preparation [56] and the maximum duration of preservation, especially for DMEK specimens [57, 58].

Described Endothelial Keratoplasty Surgical Techniques

EK is a form of corneal transplantation in which selective replacement of diseased corneal endothelium is achieved. The donor corneal endothelium is transplanted onto a carrier consisting of DM and posterior corneal stroma when the technique is DSEK (fig. 5) or without a carrier in DMEK. A variety of techniques have been used to achieve this selective replacement of diseased corneal endothelium, but this chapter will primarily focus in the DMEK surgical technique and its results and complications.

Among the different techniques for lamellar EK [59], DMEK has clinically demonstrated its superiority in terms of the visual outcome [60], visual recovery period [61], induction of posterior corneal higher-order aberrations and visual distortions [62], and risk of immunologic graft rejection [63–65]. However, widespread use of DMEK is still limited because of the challenges related to obtaining a viable donor endothelium-DM (EDM) graft and its manipulation in the AC. Moreover, the number of air-gas reinjections and associated potential complications is still higher than with other more commonly used techniques, such as DSAEK [59, 66]. This is why some hybrid techniques have been trying to combine the advantages of both, or the ease of manipulation of DSAEK and the visual outcomes of DMEK. Examples of those techniques, together with so-called ultrathin DSAEK [67], are the techniques proposed by Studeny [68], Price [69–71] and Busin [72, 73].

Stepwise techniques for graft preparation and atraumatic introduction of the EDM into the AC have been described, but 2 factors remain of significant concern: first, the intraocular manipulation time for EDM and consequent potential damage to the endothelium, and second, the postoperative rebubbling rate [74]. With the goal of improving these two factors, Güell and coworkers proposed a novel surgical approach [75] that is included in the following technique description.

Descemet Membrane Endothelial Keratoplasty Surgical Technique

Donor Preparation

Donor EDM grafts are usually prepared using the stepwise technique described by Kruse et al. [74]. Briefly, the corneoscleral button is mounted onto an 8-mm Barron Vacuum Corneal Punch (Katena, Inc, Denville, N.J., USA), marked, and stained with 0.06% trypan blue (Vision Blue; DORC, Zuidland, The Netherlands). A narrow strip of peripheral EDM is removed about 1–1.5 mm outside the 8-mm mark using a 45° blade (Alcon Laboratories, Inc, Fort Worth, T.X., USA). The central margin is then lifted and peeled off using nontoothed forceps. Our favorite approach is a single forceps approach, which has a broad base of contact that diminishes the possibility of tears (Asico AE-4359SP). Finally, the EDM is cut with an 8-mm punch (this is the most common diameter, although this is obviously individually decided, depending on the case characteristics), and the EDM graft is removed with our special forceps. To allow for better visualization of the margin, the EDM lenticule is additionally stained with 0.06% trypan blue, introduced with our forceps and manipulated with a 23G silicone-tip cannula (Canula FLEX tip 25 Ga. Edical Mix. Ref. 3221) into a 1.8-mm injector cartridge (Medicel visco-

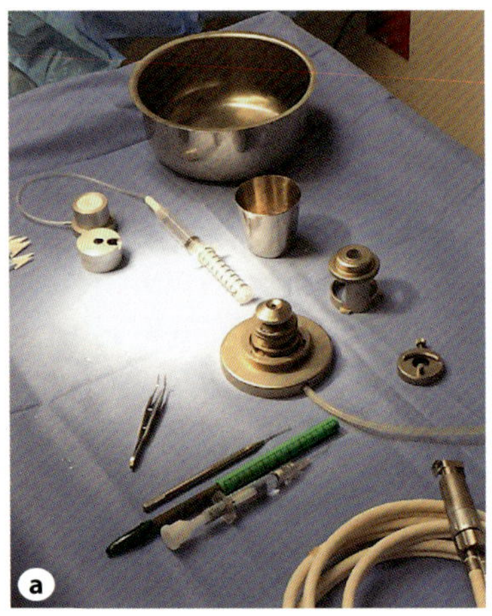 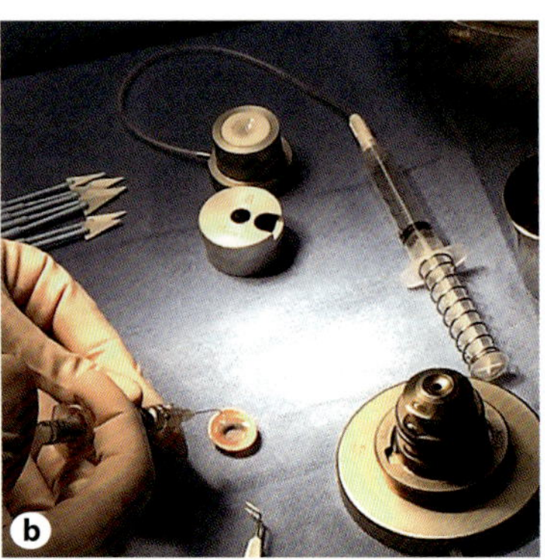 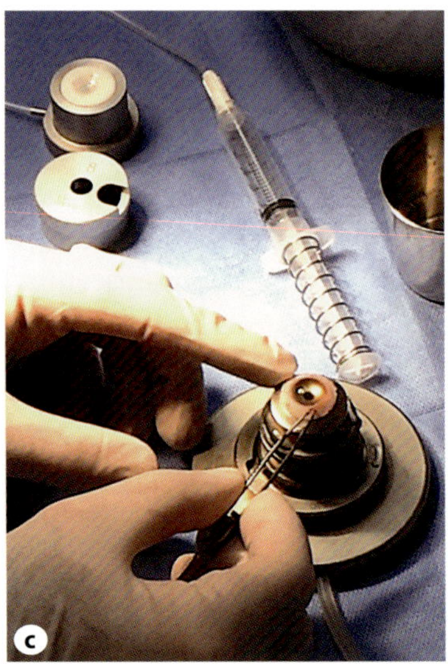

Fig. 5. Courtesy of Dr. Sadeer Hannush and Dr. Lorena Riveroll, Wills Eye Institute, Philadelphia. **a** The donor preparation table, including the artificial anterior chamber (AC), microkeratome, punch block and trephine, and viscoelastic material; a marking pen; and an S marker. **b** Placement of the viscoelastic material on the endothelial side of the donor corneoscleral tissue. **c** Mounting of the donor corneoscleral tissue on the artificial chamber, endothelial side down. **d** A modified Carriazo-Barraquer microkeratome with a 300-μm head (Moria) initiating the pass through the donor cornea mounted on the artificial AC. **e** A modified Carriazo-Barraquer microkeratome with a 300-μm head (Moria) completing a pass through the donor cornea mounted on the artificial AC. **f** Demonstration of the 300-μm cap removed with the microkeratome. **g** A gentian violet pen is used to mark the edges of the donor cornea's stromal bed in addition to S mark placement after removal of the 300-μm cap with the microkeratome. **h** Donor corneoscleral rim on a punch block after removal of the 300-μm cap. **i** An 8.5-mm trephine punching the donor cornea from the endothelial side (Katena). **j** The posterior lamellar graft after being punched to size in the well of the punch block. Note the inverted S marks. **k** The posterior lamellar graft after being punched to size in the well of the punch block (Moria). **l** Scoring the DM with a reverse Sinskey hook (over viscoelastic material or air or with a chamber maintainer connected to irrigation). **m** Stripping the DM. **n** Reverse Utrata forceps peeling the DM off the posterior surface of the host cornea. Note the edges of the epitheliectomy, performed to remove the edematous epithelium in this patient with Fuchs' dystrophy, allowing for better visualization of the AC and aiding in quicker visual rehabilitation. Additionally, note the anterior capsulorhexis with an in-the-bag intraocular lens implant. **o** The DM on the surface of the eye before being sent to pathology. **p** Mounting the donor posterior lamellar graft on the platform of the Neusidl Corneal Inserter (NCI). **q** The donor graft on the platform of the NCI, endothelial side up. **r** The donor graft rolled and retracted into the lumen of the NCI. **s** The donor graft being delivered into the AC with the NCI. **t** Unrolling of the donor graft in the AC after complete deployment of the NCI. **u** Placement of the donor posterior lamellar graft on the platform of the Busin glide with some viscoelastic material. **v** A micro-forceps pulling the donor button into the nose of the Busin glide in preparation for insertion into the eye. **w** A micro-forceps reaching across the AC to grasp the donor button; to roll it into the nose of the Busin glide, endothelial side down; and to deliver it into the eye. **x** After delivery of the donor graft from the Busin glide into the AC, the forceps are released and removed from the eye (note the position of the AC maintainer). **y** Positioning the posterior lamellar graft on the posterior host corneal surface over a small AC bubble. **z** After the lamellar graft is centered on the posterior surface of the host cornea, the AC is filled with air, and the intraocular pressure is raised above 30 mm Hg to create effective tamponade. **aa** After a period of graft tamponade with an air-filled AC, the air bubble is reduced to a diameter roughly equal to that of the graft and left in place. **bb** One day post-Descemet's stripping automated endothelial keratoplasty (EK). **cc** One month post-Descemet's stripping automated EK.

(For figure see next pages.)

   Güell · El Husseiny · Morral · Gris · Felicidad

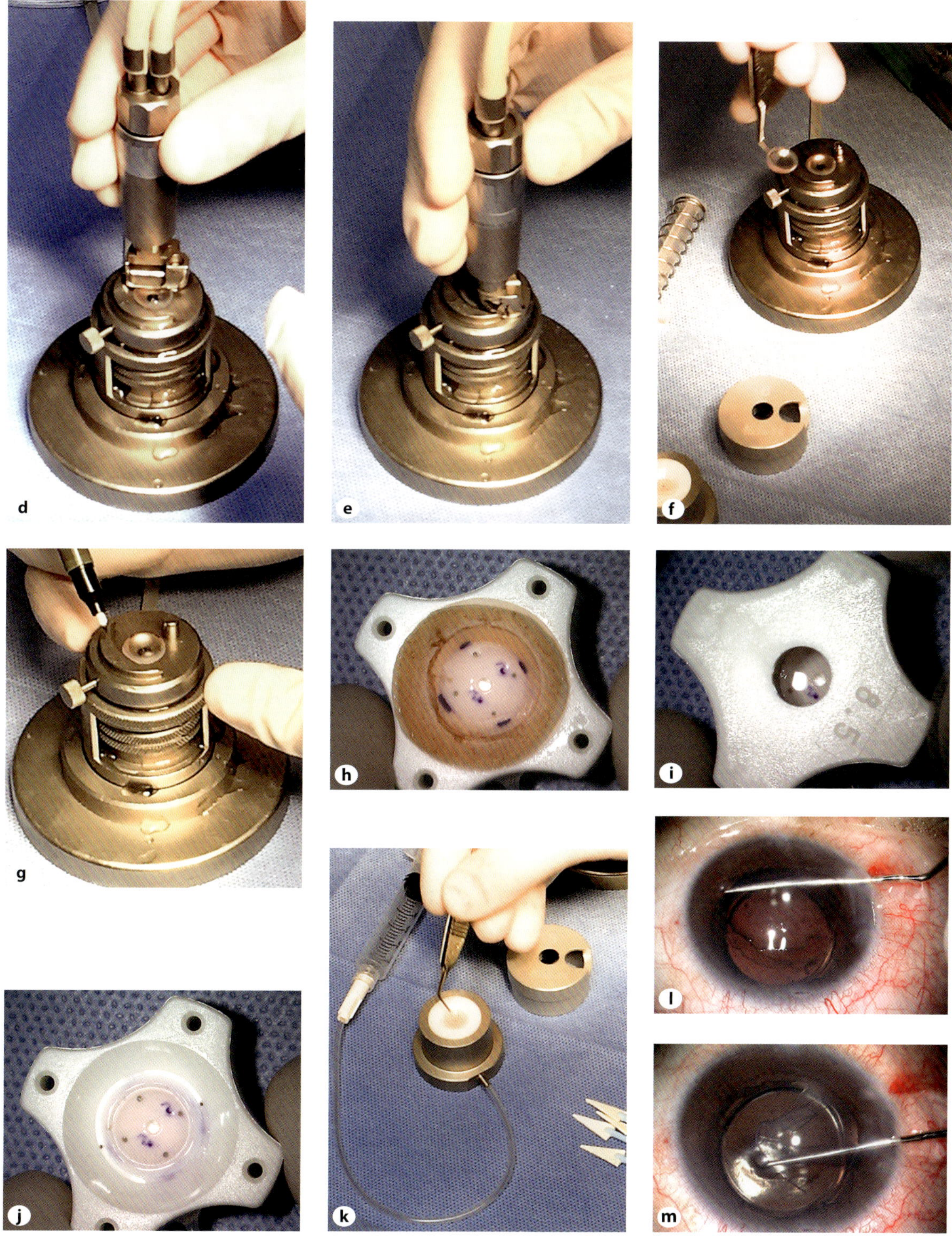

8.5

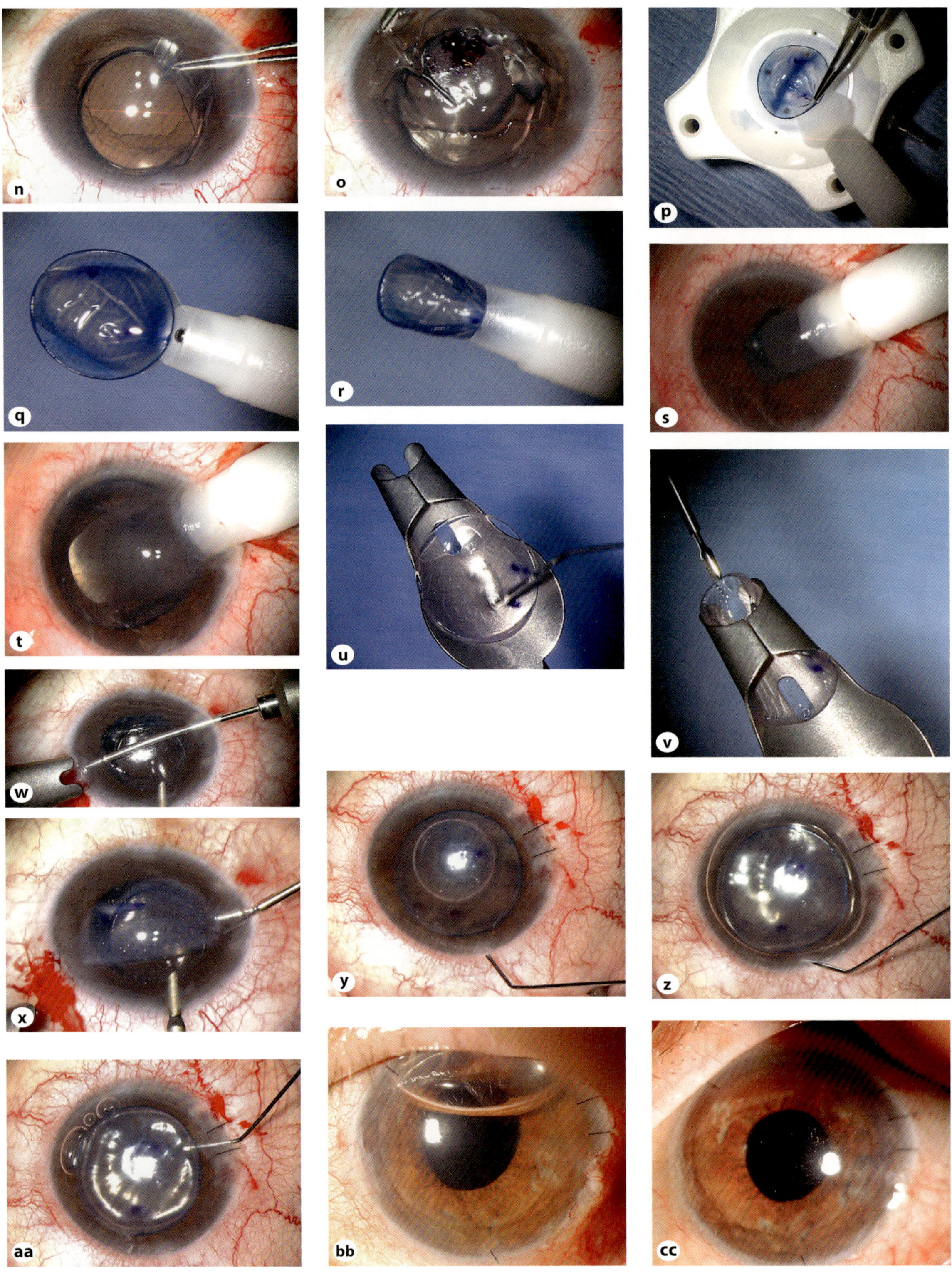

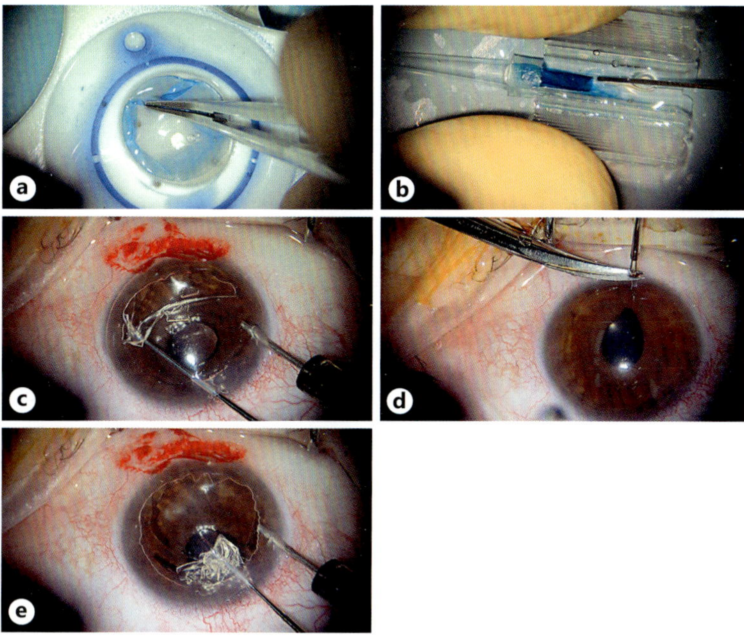

Fig. 6. a Donor and recipient preparation. The corneoscleral button is mounted onto an 8-mm Barron vacuum corneal punch and is stained with trypan blue (0.06% solution). The central margin of the EDM is lifted and peeled off using our special nontoothed wide forceps. The EDM is cut with an 8-mm punch, and the EDM graft is removed by our forceps. **b** The EDM roll is introduced into a 1.8-mm injector cartridge, which is fully filled with balanced salt solution. **c, d, e** A 25 G beveled-tip infusion cannula is inserted through one of the 2 paracenteses, and the AC is filled with air at an intraocular pressure of 20 mm Hg. A central 9-mm descemetorhexis is performed with a reverse Sinskey hook, and the recipient's DM is removed through the 2.4-mm clear corneal incision. Inferior peripheral small iridectomy is performed either through a paracentesis or with the vitrector through the main incision.

JECT; Medicel AG, Wolfhalden, Switzerland) fully filled with balanced salt solution (Alcon Laboratories, Inc) and a small air bubble in the rear part of the EDM roll in order to separate the end of the roll from the plugger. No viscoelastic material is used because it may decrease the attachment of the EDM graft (fig. 6a–c).

Recipient Preparation

Under retrobulbar anesthesia, 2 lateral 25G paracenteses are created at 2 and 10 o'clock. Through the paracentesis located on the left-hand side, a 25G beveled-tip infusion cannula (Alcon Laboratories, Inc) is inserted. A central 9- to 10-mm descemetorhexis is performed under air (infusion pressure of 20 mm Hg) with a reverse Sinskey hook (Price Endothelial Keratoplasty Hook; Moria SA, France) introduced through the other paracentesis. The recipient's DM is removed through a superior, 2.4-mm, posterior clear cor-

neal incision. All cases undergo either intraoperative inferior iridectomy using vitreoretinal forceps (Alcon/Grieshaber; advanced DSP tip ILM 23 Ga. Forceps Ref. 723.44 and Holder Ref. 712.0041) through a 20G inferior paracentesis or preoperative ND:YAG laser inferior iridotomy (fig. 6d–f).

Donor Endothelium-Descemet Membrane Insertion and Positioning

The most challenging step of DMEK is the insertion of the EDM graft while maintaining the adequate orientation and its subsequent attachment to the recipient's corneal stroma. First, after lowering the pressure of the irrigation fluid to an intraocular pressure (IOP) of 5 mm Hg, the EDM roll is gently injected, with the main incision completely occluded by the tip of the injector. The 25G infusion cannula is withdrawn just before the injector is retracted from the main incision to prevent the EDM roll from sweeping through the main incision. Next, the 2.4-mm incision is closed with 1 or 2 interrupted 10.0 nylon sutures to ensure that the main incision is reasonably watertight. Then, a Gills cannula connected to an automated irrigation aspiration system (Constellation, Alcon Laboratories, Inc) is introduced through the main incision, with continuous irrigation set at 60–100 mm Hg, which is controlled by a technician through the Constellation software. However, the actual IOP is much lower because of the small caliber of the Gills cannula. Low-pressure irrigation flow is the key to centering the EDM roll, maintaining the adequate orientation of the graft, and unfolding the EDM graft. In most cases, and especially in younger donors, an air bubble is slowly injected through one of the paracenteses into the inner lumen of the EDM roll until complete unfolding is achieved, and the EDM lenticule is spread out over the iris surface. As unfolding is generally much more difficult in younger donors, higher flow pressures are often required, and the technician is asked to change the parameters set in the Constellation software. Once the air bubble occupies about two thirds of the AC, the irrigation fluid is withdrawn, and the centration and positioning are rechecked.

Finally, the air bubble between the recipient's cornea and the graft is completely removed. Attachment of the graft to the recipient's posterior corneal stroma is achieved by injection of air mixed with 20% sulfur hexafluoride (SF_6) gas (the maximum nonexpansile concentration) underneath the EDM lenticule from the center of the pupil, until the AC is almost fully filled, leaving only a 0.5-mm peripheral meniscus (fig. 7).

In most cases, we use a very low infusion pressure during the AC manipulations, and, once the graft is adequately centered, with a relatively empty AC and soft eye, we finish the peripheral opening of the membrane with soft touches over the corneal epithelium (fig. 8).

With this approach, we do not need to inject air over the membrane, and we can directly inject the 20% SF_6 underneath it from the center of the pupil to position the membrane against the recipient stroma, again reducing the total manipulation time.

Postoperative Management
Patients are examined immediately and 1–2 hours, 24 hours, 1 week, 3 weeks, 2.4 months and 6 months after the surgery. Postoperative standard treatment consists of 0.3% topical tobramycin and 0.1% dexamethasone (Tobradex; Alcon Cusi, El Masnou, Barcelona, Spain) 4 times daily for 3 weeks and 2 times daily for the following 8 weeks; 0.5% timolol (Cusimolol; Alcon Cusi) 2 times daily for 12 weeks; and 0.05% dexamethasone and 1% chloramphenicol ointment (Deicol; Alcon Cusi) at bedtime for 2–3 months, or stopped in the absence of any inflammatory signs or signs of rejection.

Given no contraindications, oral methylprednisolone (Urbason, Sanofi-Aventis Pharma SA, Barcelona, Spain) is also prescribed and slowly tapered for the first 3 weeks, as follows: 40 mg/day for 3 days, 20 mg/day for 3 more days, 10 mg/day for 1 week, and 10 mg every 48 hours for 1 week.

As 20% SF_6 is progressively reabsorbed after the surgery (generally, SF_6 occupies about three fourths of the AC 1 day postoperatively and about one half of the AC 5 days postoperatively), patients are instructed to lie in the supine face-up position for periods of 15 minutes, for 2 hours total, in the morning and in the afternoon, with 3 different head inclinations during the first week: with the chin close to the chest, with the chin parallel to the floor, or with the head hanging backward slightly. The goal is to use the air-gas bubble as a tamponade over the whole lenticule surface (fig. 9).

Published Outcomes of Endothelial Keratoplasty

The updated outcomes of the two main surgical approaches, or DSAEK and DMEK, are summarized in tables 1 and 2.

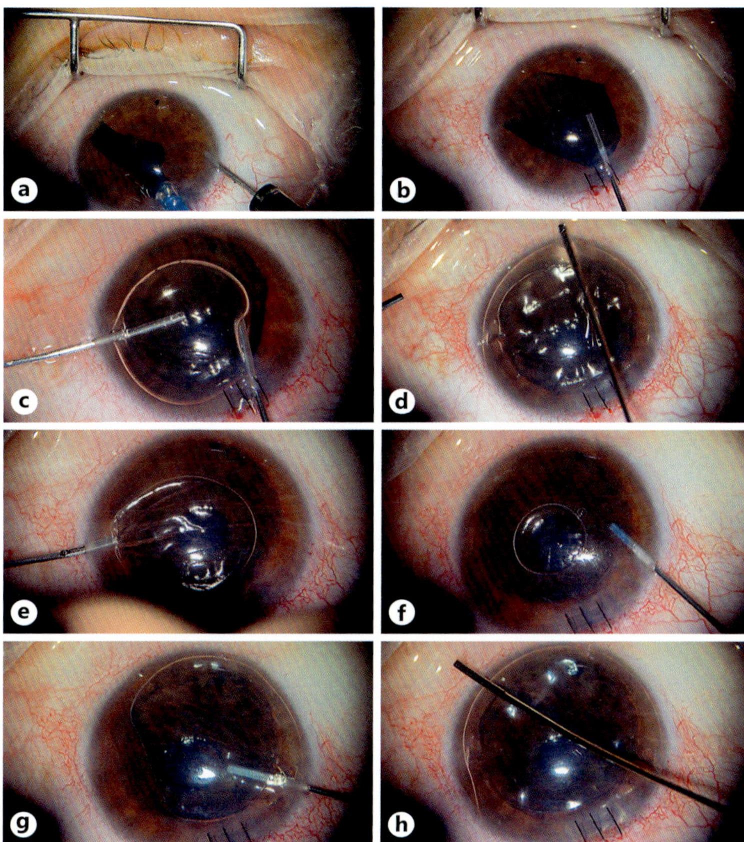

Fig. 7. Donor EDM insertion and positioning. **a** The pressure of the irrigation fluid in the AC is lowered to an intraocular pressure of 5 mm Hg, and the EDM roll is gently injected into the AC. **b**, **c** A Gills or a hydrodissection cannula connected to the automated irrigation aspiration system is introduced through the main incision, with low irrigation fluid flow, and the EDM roll is centered. **d–f** The EDM graft is unfolded by insertion of an air bubble into the inner lumen of the EDM roll. Then, air is slowly injected, and the unfolded EDM lenticule is spread out over the iris surface. Once the centration and positioning are rechecked, the air bubble between the recipient cornea and the graft is completely removed. **g**, **h** Attachment of the graft to the recipient's posterior corneal stroma is achieved by injection of 20% sulfur hexafluoride (SF_6) gas underneath the EDM lenticule from the center of the pupil, until the AC is completely filled.

Comments about the Descemet Membrane Endothelial Keratoplasty Technique

The degree of visual recovery is generally so good after DMEK that most consider surgery much earlier than before with other techniques (sometimes in FECD patients with 20/20 vision but fluctuations during the daytime) and consider the second eye surgery much sooner than before, as if it were a cataract surgery case [76]. From a refractive point of view, you should expect a very low hyperopic shift related to the progressive postoperative corneal thinning [77], and sometimes, lower vision than expected might be related to some residual irregular astigmatism due to the long-standing corneal edema, which is correctable with rigid gas-permeable contact lenses [78, 79].

Different techniques for graft preparation and atraumatic introduction of a graft have been described and have been really perfected, but unfolding and positioning the EDM roll once introduced into the AC is one of the most challenging steps of DMEK surgery and may require longer operating times and various attempts that may result in increased endothelial cell loss. Moreover, inadequate positioning of the membrane over the host stroma, with folds and/or striae, is quite frequent, with an associated higher graft detachment rate postoperatively [74, 80].

Therefore, our group developed a new bimanual infusion technique that successfully achieved insertion and proper positioning of EDM grafts, with a brief intraocular manipulation time and a low postoperative rebubbling rate, regardless of

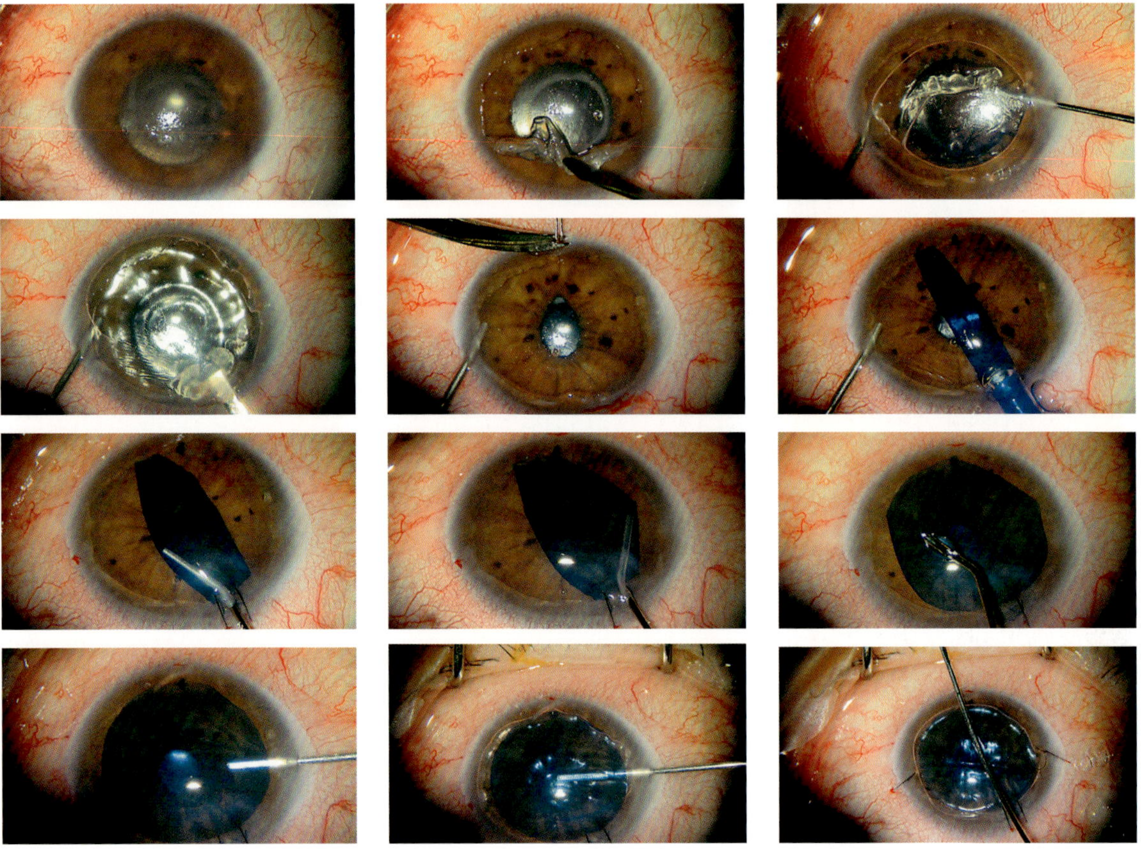

Fig. 8. Advanced technique. The donor preparation is the same as with our standard technique, with a wide desce-metorhexis and peripheral iridectomy under pressure-controlled irrigation through our 25G cannula. Introduction of the roll under 5 mm Hg of infusion pressure is also the same, but in this approach, we do not inject air, but rather liquid, under low-pressure-controlled infusion. Once the positioning of the membrane (sometimes with some external point pressure over the cornea) over the iris is acceptable, we inject gas underneath the membrane, pushing it over the recipient stroma.

the preservation method and the donor's age [75].

In our study, the visual outcome was similar to that in previously published series, with 40% of eyes achieving 20/20 or better vision initially and 86% of eyes achieving 20/30 or better vision at 6 months [30, 61, 71, 81–84].

The fact that the EDM graft was smaller (8 mm) than the recipient's descemetorhexis (9–10 mm) did not affect the final visual outcome, but mild peripheral corneal edema was occasionally observed at the junction of the EDM graft and the bare stroma, which produced transient symptoms of foreign-body sensation in some cases. In any case, we thought that this difference in size would allow a better attachment rate, as has also been recently suggested by the Kruse group [85].

We think that the key advantage was that the infusion cannula, which was at a controlled pressure, maintained a constant low IOP and prevented the AC from collapsing during the unrolling and positioning maneuvers. In fact, in most cases, positioning of the membrane over the iris during

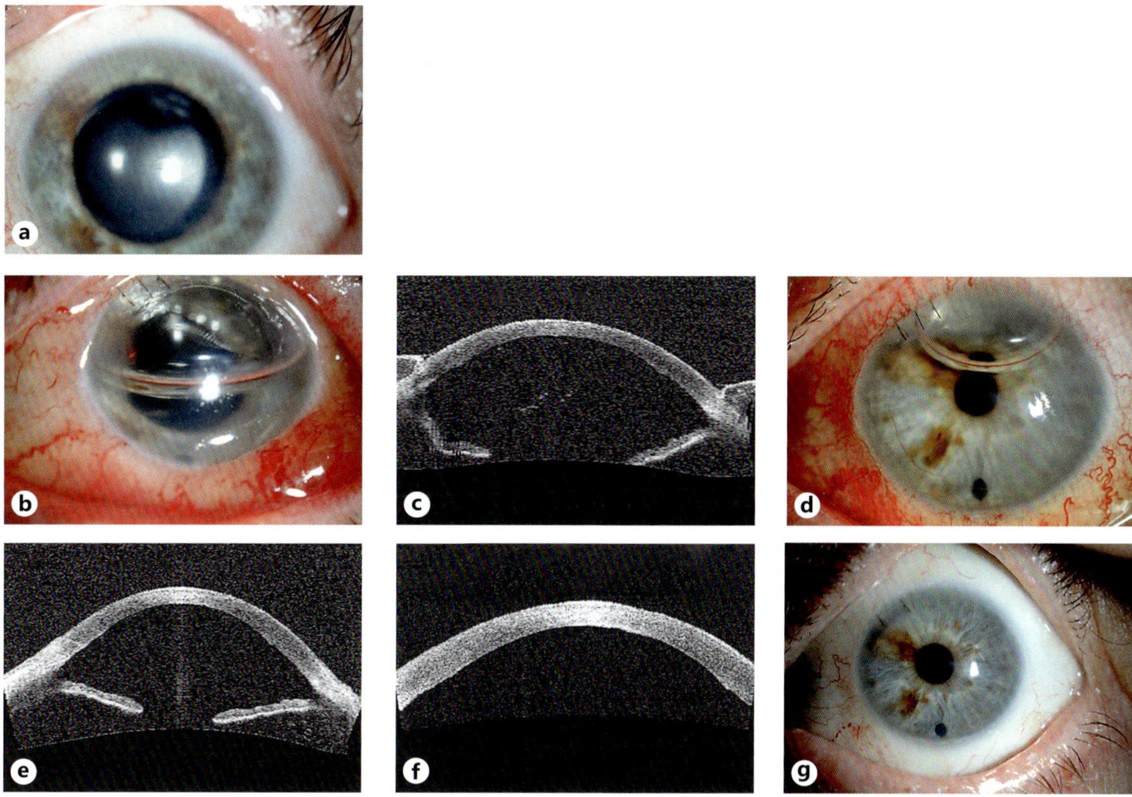

Fig. 9. A 62-year-old woman with Fuchs' endothelial dystrophy and mild pseudophakic corneal edema underwent DM EK (DMEK). **a** Preoperative clinical photography shows guttae, pigmentary deposits on the corneal endothelium, and a well-centered intraocular lens in the capsular sac. The best spectacle-corrected visual acuity was 20/50. **b** Visante™ optical coherence tomography (OCT) (Carl Zeiss Meditec, Jena, Germany), with a preoperative image showing mild corneal edema. **c** Tamponade is achieved with 20% SF_6. One day after DMEK, the 20% SF_6 bubble occupies two thirds of the AC. **d** Two days after DMEK, partial reabsorption of the 20% SF_6 occurs, and the 20% SF_6 bubble occupies one half of the AC. **e, f** One week after surgery, total reabsorption of the gas bubble is noted. Visante OCT (**f**) shows complete attachment of the EDM graft. No reinjections are required. **g, h** Three months after surgery. **g** Clinical photograph shows a clear cornea with a completely attached EDM graft. **h** A Visante OCT image shows complete attachment of the EDM graft. The best spectacle-corrected visual acuity had increased to 20/20. No episodes of immunologic rejection were documented.

infusion was good enough to avoid the injection of air over the membrane, instead occurring directly underneath to push up the membrane into its final position. As we previously mentioned, with touches over the cornea, we sometimes completely unfolded the peripheral edges of the membrane, and the number of cases in which we needed air over the membrane was significantly reduced. Moreover, adequate orientation and centration of the graft was easily monitored because trypan blue staining was visible throughout the procedure, despite the cloudiness of the anterior host stroma. Obviously, if visualization is difficult, we can always use an endolight probe (fig. 10), although some other more sophisticated strategies have also been described, such as the use of optical coherence tomography [60] or the use of a handheld slit beam [86].

Table 1. DMEK update

Author	Publication	Year	Eyes	Study	Follow-up, months	Rebubbling for dislocation, %	Primary graft failure, %	Graft rejection, %	Refractive astigmat	SE	ECC loss, %	Mean BSCVA
Price	Ophthalmology	2009	60		3	63	8		0.9	0.49	30	
Droutsas	Klin Monbl Augen	2010	78		6						31.50	
Dapena	Arch Soc Esp Oftal	2011	120		6						32.18	
Anshu	Ophthalmology	2012	141		13			0.70				
Yoerkuel	Klin Monbl Augen	2012	75		12.1	31						0.5
Laaser	Am J Ophthalmol	2012	61	DMEK + cataract	6				−1.5	0.9	39.70	20/30
Güell	Cornea	2013	15	bimanual technique	6	6.60		0			26	
Van Dijt	Cont Lens Ant eye	2013	300		6	10				0.33	34.60	
Droutsas	Cornea	2013	25	begining surgeon	6	36	4				45.40	
Gorovoy	Cornea	2014	75	complications	3	2.60	2.60					20/25
Chaurasia	Ophthalmology	2014	492	pseudophakic	6	30	3.10				26	20/25
Güell	Current series	2014	138		24	1.44	0.72	0	0.2		28	20/30

Kruse et al. [74] described that turning of tightly rolled EDMs required filling the AC with fluid and then placing small jets of fluid next to the roll. In some cases, rolls that did not form required direct EDM contact with a cannula, which may induce trauma to the endothelium. None of these maneuvers was required in our bimanual infusion technique, as easy manipulation and positioning could be achieved for both fresh and cultured tissue, even in tightly rolled EDMs (younger donors). However, the mean cell loss (26 ± 20%) was similar to that in previous studies [30, 31, 61, 83], although, as it has already been reported, this loss might be overestimated [71].

The most frequent complication of DMEK surgery is incomplete attachment of the graft in the early postoperative course [87].

DMEK started out with air reinjection rates ranging from 50 to 77% [30, 61, 83], but most experienced centers are currently reporting rates of 0–20% [28, 71, 82]. Dapena et al. [88] reported 15/120 eyes (18%) with graft detachment (10 complete and 5 partial), with 11/120 eyes progressing to graft failure and needing repeat surgery, and usually DSEK. In another study of 135 eyes, Dapena et al. [82] found that with surgical experience, graft detachment rates decreased to 4.4%, but no correlation with clinical outcomes (best spectacle-corrected visual acuity and central enhanced corneal compensation) was noted. Laaser et al. [89] reported that a significantly higher number of air injections was necessary for Optisol GS-stored grafts (34/36 eyes, 92%) compared with outer cornea donors (26/45 eyes, 58%) (p < 0.05).

Intracameral injection of 20% SF$_6$ had already been used to treat DM detachments [90, 91]. In our opinion, tamponade with 20% SF$_6$ as well as a very regular apposition of the membrane over the host stroma and postoperative head positioning are the key factors explaining the low rebubbling rate found in our published preliminary study (6.6%). In fact, in our experience over the

Table 2. DSEK/DSAEK

Author	Publication	Year	N	Keratoplasty	Follow-up, months	Graft survival, %	Primary graft failure, %	Graft rejection, %	Dislocation, %	Astigmat D	ECC loss, %	BSCVA, mean
Price	J Refract Surg	2005	50	DSEK	6		6			1.5		≥20/40, 62%
Price	Ophthalmology	2006	216	DSEK microk vs. manual	6		7		8	1.5		≥20/40, 69%
Koening	Ophthalmology	2007	26	DSAEK	3		3	12	35			20/45
Koening	Cornea	2007	34	DSAEK	6		3	18	26.50		50	20/42
Price	Am J Ophthalmol	2008	40	DSAEK. Precut vs. diss	12	100	0	5	10		34	≥20/40, 80%
Bahar	Ophthalmology	2008	16	DSEK-DSAEK-PK-DLEK	12	98	2	2	15	1.4 DSAEK 3.8 PK	40	20/44
Chen	Cornea	2008	100	DSAEK	6		0		3	1.2		≥20/40, 81%
Basak	Indian J Ophtahlmol	2008	75	DSAEK	3		1	1	8	1.1	27	≥20/60, 82,7%
Bahar	Am J Ophthalmol	2009	26	DSAEK guide vs. forceps	6		3	3	8/19	2.2, 1.3	25, 34	20/37, 20/42
Terry	Ophthalmology	2009	225	DSAEK + CAT	12		0.30		3	1.1	31	≥20/40, 80%
Jun	Cornea	2009	45	DSAEK	5							
Terry	Ophthalmology	2009	100	DSAEK. precut	12	100	0		1	0.09	29	≥20/40, 92%
Ahmed	Am J Ophthalmol	2010	44	DSEK	12		2.20					20/29
Weller	Klin Monbl Augen	2010	28	DSEK	12		10.70			1.4	28	0.4 log MAR
Price	Ophthalmology	2011	165	DSEK	60	95	6	1.20			53	
Villarrubia	Arch Soc Esp Oftal	2011	75	DSAEK	36	97.50	6.50	1.30	22.50		42	
Chaurasia	Br J Ophthalmol	2011	309	DSEK	12				8.70			
Van der Meulen	Cornea	2012	34	DSEK	64							0.33 LogMAR
Ang	Clin Ophthalmol	2012	68	DSAEK	12		3	1.50	0	1.7	22.40	0.27 LogMAR
Li	Ophthalmology	2012	108	DSAEK	36							≥20/25:70.4%
Phillips	Cornea	2012	100	DSAEK	6		0		2		16	20/35
Khor	Am J Ophthalmol	2013	100	DSAEK	12		1	2.60	2		14.90	≥20/40, 50%
Busin	Ophthalmology	2013	285	DSAEK ultrathin	24		2.80	3.30	3.90		36.60	≥20/20, 48.8%
Price	Ophthalmology	2013	173	DSAEK	36	96	4	9			52	
Moura	Arg Bras Oftalmol	2013	65	DSEK				15.30	21.50			
Basak	Indian J Ophtahlmol	2013	430	DSEK	18.7		3.30	1.20	4.90		54.20	
Kosker	Cornea	2013	30	DSEK vs. PK	24			13.3 vs. 333		1.05 vs. 3.57 D		0,23 LogMAR
Nakagawa	Am J Ophthalmol	2014	134	DSAEK precut	36			2.20	8.90		51	0,22 LogMAR

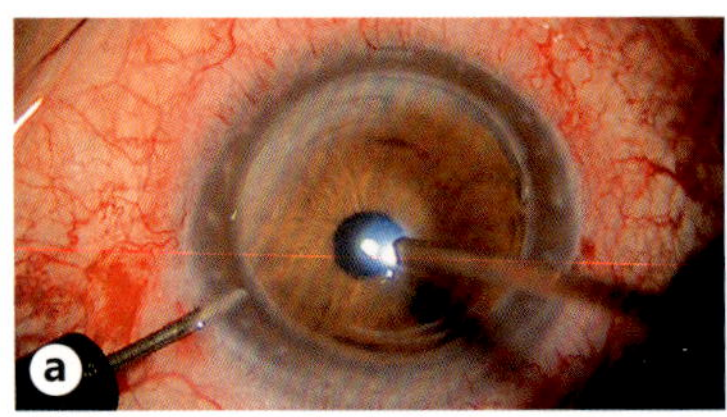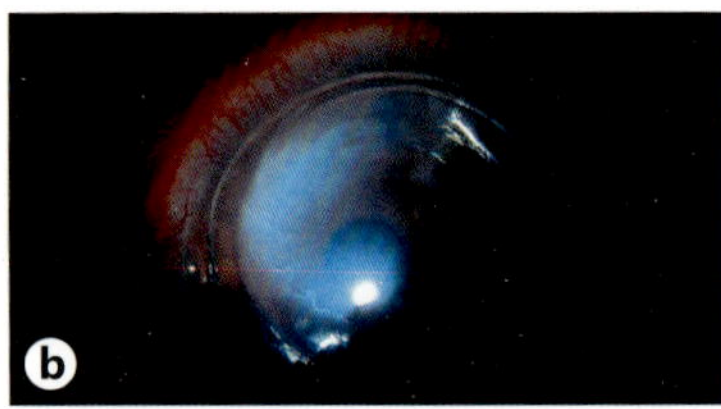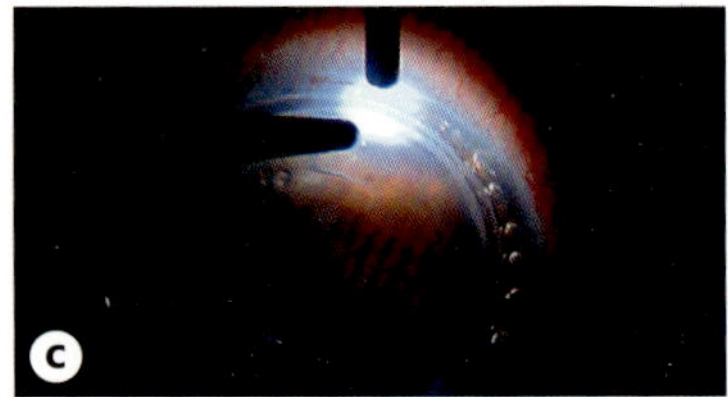

Fig. 10. The endoillumination probe can be easily used during surgery either to visualize any vitreous strands (**a**) or to visualize, in the case of corneal stromal edema and/or opacities, the DM (**b, c**) during DMEK.

last 3 years, the rate of rebubbling dropped to less than 1%. Thompson [92] studied the kinetics of intraocular gases and found that the half-life of air was 1.6/0.9 days in phakic/aphakic eyes, that the half-life of 20% SF$_6$ was 2.8/2.4 days in phakic/aphakic eyes, and that the half-life of 10% perfluoropropane was 5.7/4.5 days in phakic/aphakic eyes. As most cases of EDM graft detachments occur within the first 24–72 hours, we chose to use 20% SF$_6$ instead of air to ensure proper tamponade during this critical period. Moreover, head positioning provides a tamponade effect in all areas of the EDM graft, even when the gas only partially occupies the AC. Although some authors suggest that adherence of the donor issue to the posterior stroma is achieved only if a tamponade effect is obtained at a relatively high pressure, our experience does not support this statement, as complete attachment of the EDM graft was achieved even though high IOP was not reached at any time. Most cases were even slightly hypotonic during the first 24 hours. In our opinion, it is the longer persistence of SF$_6$, instead of high IOP, that leads to complete adherence of the EDM graft. This issue, however, remains controversial between different study groups.

Decreasing the rebubbling rate has many advantages, which include avoiding further endothelial damage, avoiding complications related to air reinjection (infection, inflammation, acute glaucoma, IOP spikes, etc.) and reducing inconvenience for patients compared to requiring 1 week of positioning and prohibiting taking an airplane for 2 or 3 days. With respect to complications, prolonged contact of gas with the corneal endothelium in aphakic eyes can lead to corneal decompensation, but no toxicity to the endothelium has been described with short-term use [93]. Although we could not demonstrate a decrease in the damage to the endothelium with our surgical approach, we do not think that 20% SF$_6$ caused any toxicity, as it was completely reabsorbed within the first week after the surgery in most cases. A controlled study comparing 20% SF$_6$ tamponade to air alone would clarify this phenomenon, and this is the study that we are conducting at our center.

Another potential complication associated with SF$_6$ is the increase in IOP in the early postoperative period [94]. Chen and Thompson [95] demonstrated a 43% incidence of IOP elevation greater than 25 mm Hg, with most of the cases occurring within the first 24 hours after pars plana vitrectomy. Spikes in IOP have been described for both 20% SF$_6$ and 10% perfluoropropane, but we prefer to use 20% SF$_6$, as the incidence is much lower. Additionally, inferior iridectomy/iridotomy should always be performed to avoid pupillary block glaucoma. With minimal-sized iridectomy/iridotomy, none of our patients perceived uniocular polyopia or glare, and no IOP spike in the immediate postoperative period was encountered in our study group or in our later experience.

In conclusion, from our point of view, DMEK is the best technique for endothelial transplantation. The particular surgical approaches and strategies should be properly described and controlled over time in order to gain consensus on the best ones. Additionally, as we mentioned earlier in this chapter, DSAEK (especially the so-called 'ultrathin' techniques) and, in particular circumstances, PKP, should be included in our surgical armamentarium because they will be more appropriate for some surgeons in selected cases [96]. Although most of us prefer to perform DMEK on uncomplicated pseudophakic eyes, the triple procedure is also commonly performed worldwide [97], and we already know that cataract surgery after DMEK can be successfully performed, with no increased risk of detachment [98]. Additionally, DMEK is becoming the technique of choice when endothelial transplantation is needed after failed PKP or DSAEK [99].

References

1 Edelhauser HF: The balance between corneal transparency and edema: the Proctor Lecture. Invest Ophthalmol Vis Sci 2006;47:1755–1767.
2 Robbins and Cotran pathologic basis of disease. 7th ed. / [edited by] Vinay Kumar, Abul K. Abbas, Nelson Fausto ; with illustrations by James A. Perkins. Philadelphia : Elsevier Saunders, c2005. xv, 1525 p. ill. (chiefly col.) ; 29 cm. + 1 CD-ROM (4 3/4 in.) RB111.R62, 2005 ISBN: 0721601871.
3 Bourne RR, Minassian DC, Dart JK, et al: Effect of cataract surgery on the corneal endothelium: modern phacoemulsification compared with extracapsular cataract surgery. Ophthalmology 2004; 111:679–685.
4 Joyce NC: Proliferative capacity of the corneal endothelium. Prog Retin Eye Res 2003;22:359–389.
5 Fuchs E: Dystrophia epithelialis corneae. Graefes Arch Clin Exp Ophthalmol 1910;76:478–508.
6 Krachmer JH, Purcell JJ Jr, Young CW, et al: Corneal endothelial dystrophy: a study of 64 families. Arch Ophthalmol 1978;96:2036–2039.
7 Adamis AP, Filatov V, Tripathi BJ, et al: Fuchs' endothelial dystrophy of the cornea. Surv Ophthalmol 1993;38:149–168.
8 Borboli S, Colby K: Mechanisms of disease: Fuchs' endothelial dystrophy. Ophthalmol Clin North Am 2002;15:17–25.
9 Biswas S, Munier FL, Yardley J, et al: Missense mutations in COL8A2, the gene encoding the alpha2 chain of type VIII collagen, cause two forms of corneal endothelial dystrophy. Hum Mol Genet 2001;10:2415–2423.
10 Cross HE, Maumenee AE, Cantolino SJ: Inheritance of Fuchs' endothelial dystrophy. Arch Ophthalmol 1971;85:268–272.

11 Maurice DM: The cornea and sclera; in Davson H (ed): The Eye. New York, Academic Press, 1984.
12 Seitzman GD, Gottsch JD, Stark WJ: Cataract surgery in patients with Fuchs' corneal dystrophy: expanding recommendations for cataract surgery without simultaneous keratoplasty. Ophthalmology 2005;112:441–446.
13 Corneal endothelial photography. American Academy of Ophthalmology. Ophthalmology 1991;98:1464–1468.
14 Mamalis N, Edelhauser HF, Dawson DG, et al: Toxic anterior segment syndrome. J Cataract Refractive Surg 2006;32:324–333.
15 Jehan FS, Mamalis N, Spencer TS, et al: Postoperative sterile endophthalmitis (TASS) associated with the memory lens. J Cataract Refract Surg 2000;26: 1773–1777.
16 Parihk CH, Edelhauser HF: Ocular surgical pharmacology: corneal endothelial safety and toxicity. Curr Opin Ophthalmol 2003;14:178–185.
17 Moshirfar M, Whitehead G, Beutler BC, et al: Toxic anterior segment syndrome after Verisyse iris-supported phakic intraocular lens implantation. J Cataract Refract Surg 2006;32:1233–1237.
18 Tillett CW: Posterior lamellar keratoplasty. Am J Ophthalmol 1956;41:530–533.
19 Barraquer JI: Lamellar keratoplasty. (Special techniques). Ann Ophthalmol 1972;4:437–469.
20 Busin M, Arffa RC, Sebastiani A: Endokeratoplasty as an alternative to penetrating keratoplasty for the surgical treatment of diseased endothelium: initial results. Ophthalmology 2000;107:2077–2082.
21 Güell JL, Gris O, Guerrero E, et al: Preliminary results with posterior lamellar keratoplasty for endothelial failure. Br J Ophthalmol 2003;87:241–243.

22 Melles GR, Eggink FA, Lander F, et al: A surgical technique for posterior lamellar keratoplasty. Cornea 1998;17:618–626.
23 Melles GR, Lander F, van Dooren BT, et al: Preliminary clinical results of posterior lamellar keratoplasty through a sclerocorneal pocket incision. Ophthalmology 2000;107:1850–1856; discussion 1857.
24 Giebel AW: DMEK: where less is more. Int Ophthalmol Clin 2013;53:1–14.
25 Melles GRJ, Wijdh RHJ, Nieuwendaal CP: A technique to excise the Descemet membrane from a recipient cornea (descemetorhexis). Cornea 2004;23:286–288.
26 Gorovoy MS: Descemet-stripping automated endothelial keratoplasty. Cornea 2006;25:886–889.
27 Statistical Report on Eye Banking Activity for 2007.2008;1–25. Eye Bank Association of America Washington, DC.
28 Melles GR, Ong TS, Ververs B, et al: Preliminary clinical results of Descemet membrane endothelial keratoplasty. Am J Ophthalmol 2008;145:222–227.
29 Ham L, Dapena I, van Luijk C, et al: Descemet membrane endothelial keratoplasty (DMEK) for Fuchs endothelial dystrophy: review of the first 50 consecutive cases. Eye (Lond) 2009;23:1990–1998.
30 Price MO, Giebel AW, Fairchild KM, et al: Descemet's membrane endothelial keratoplasty: prospective multicenter study of visual and refractive outcomes and endothelial survival. Ophthalmology 2009;116:2361–2368.
31 Ham L, van Luijk C, Dapena I, et al: Endothelial cell density after descemet membrane endothelial keratoplasty: 1- to 2-year follow-up. Am J Ophthalmol 2009;148:521–527.

32 Koenig SB, Covert DJ, Dupps WJ Jr, et al: Visual acuity, refractive error, and endothelial cell density six months after Descemet Stripping and Automated Endothelial Keratoplasty (DSAEK). Cornea 2007;26:670–674.

33 Mearza AA, Qureshi MA, Rostron CK: Experience and 12-month results of Descemet-stripping endothelial keratoplasty (DSEK) with a small-incision technique. Cornea 2007;26:279–283.

34 Guerra FP, Arundhati A, Price MO, et al: Endothelial keratoplasty: fellow eyes comparison of Descemet stripping automated endothelial keratoplasty and Descemet membrane endothelial keratoplasty. Cornea 2011;30:1382–1386.

35 Parker J, Dirisamer M, Naveiras M, et al: Endothelial cell density after Descemet membrane endothelial keratoplasty: 1- to 4-year follow-up. Am J Ophthalmol 2011;151:1107.

36 Price MO, Price FW Jr: Endothelial cell loss after Descemet stripping with endothelial keratoplasty influencing factors and 2-year trend. Ophthalmology 2008; 115:857–865.

37 Melles GR: Posterior lamellar keratoplasty: DLEK to DSEK to DMEK. Cornea 2006;25:879–881.

38 Price MO, Price FW: Descemet's stripping endothelial keratoplasty. Curr Opin Ophthalmol 2007;18:290–294.

39 Voci E, Kelley K: From the patient's perspective; in Price FW, Price MO (eds): DSEK: What You Need to Know about Endothelial Keratoplasty. Thorofare, NJ, SLACK Inc, 2009, pp 17–23.

40 Terry MA: A new approach for endothelial transplantation: deep lamellar endothelial keratoplasty. Int Ophthalmol Clin 2003;43:183–193.

41 Price FW Jr, Price MO: Endothelial keratoplasty to restore clarity to a failed penetrating graft. Cornea 2006;25:895–899.

42 Covert DJ, Koening SB: Descemet stripping and automated endothelial keratoplasty (DSAEK) in eyes with failed penetrating keratoplasty. Cornea 2007;26: 692–696.

43 Price MO, Price FW Jr: Descemet's stripping endothelial keratoplasty for treatment of iridocorneal endothelial syndrome. Cornea 2007;26:493–497.

44 Elder MJ, Stack RR: Glove rupture following penetrating keratoplasty: how often, why, and what can we do to prevent it? Cornea 2004;23:776–780.

45 Price MO, Price FW Jr, Trespalacios R: Endothelial keratoplasty technique for aniridic aphakia eyes. J Catract Refract Sur 2007;33:376–379.

46 Suh LH, Kymionis GD, Culberston WW, et al: Descemet Stripping with endothelial Keratoplasty in aphakic eyes. Arch Ophthalmol 2008;126:268–270.

47 Macsai MS, Kara-Jose AC: Suure technique for Descemet Stripping and endothelial keratoplasty. Cornea 2007;26: 1123–1126.

48 Heindl LM, Riss S, Adler W, et al: Split cornea transplantation: relationship between storage time of split donor tissue and outcome. Ophthalmology 2013; 120:889–907.

49 Kitzmann AS, Goins KM, Reed C, et al: Eye Bank survey of surgeons using precut donor tissue for Descemet stripping automated endothelial keratoplasty. Cornea 2008;27:634–639.

50 Dupps BJ, Qian Y, Meisler DM: Multivarite model of refractive shift in Descemet-stripping automated endothelial keratoplasty. Cataract Refrac Surg 2008; 34:578–584.

51 Chen ES, Terry MA, Shamie N, et al: Precut tissue in Descemet's stripping automated endothelial keratoplasty (donor characteristics and early postoperative complications). Ophthalmology 2008;115:497–502.

52 Cheng YY, Hendrikse F, Pels E, et al: Preliminary results of femtosecond laser assisted descemet stripping endothelial keratoplasty. Arch Ophthalmol 2008; 126:1351–1356.

53 Jones YJ, Goins KM, Sutphin JE, et al: Comparison of the femtosecond laser (IntraLase) versus manual microkeratome (Moria ALTK) in dissection of the donor in endothelial keratoplasty (initial study in eye bank eyes). Cornea 2008;27: 88–93.

54 Mehta JS, Parthasarthy A, Por YM, et al: Femtosecond laser-assited endothelial keratoplasty (a laboratory model). Cornea 2008;27:706–712.

55 Price MO, Price FW: Descemet's stripping with endothelial keratoplasty (comparative outcomes with microkeratome-dissected and manually dissected donor tissue). Ophthalmology 2006;113: 1936–1942.

56 Muraine M, Gueudry J, He Z, et al: Novel technique for the preparation of corneal grafts for descemet membrane endothelial keratoplasty. Am J Ophthalmol 2013;156:851–859.

57 Feng MT, Bukhard ZN, Price FW, et al: Effect of donor preparation-to-use times on descemet membrane endothelial keratoplasty outcomes. Cornea 2013;32: 1080–1082.

58 Schlötzer-Schrehardt U, Bachmann BO, Tourtas T, et al: Reproducibility of graft preparations in Descemet's membrane endothelial keratoplasty. Ophthalmology 2013;120:1769–1777.

59 Anshu A, Price MO, Tan DT, et al: Endothelial keratoplasty: a revolution in evolution. Surv Ophthalmol 2012;57: 236–252.

60 Guerra FP, Anshu A, Price MO, et al: Endothelial keratoplasty: fellow eyes comparison of Descemet stripping automated endothelial keratoplasty and Descemet membrane endothelial keratoplasty. Cornea 2011;30:1382–1386.

61 Guerra FP, Anshu A, Price MO, et al: Descemet's membrane endothelial keratoplasty: prospective study of 1-year visual outcomes, graft survival, and endothelial cell loss. Ophthalmology 2011; 118:2368–2373.

62 Rudolph M, Laaser K, Bachmann BO, et al: Corneal higher-order aberrations after Descemet's membrane endothelial keratoplasty. Ophthalmology 2012;119: 528–535.

63 Anshu A, Price MO, Price FW Jr: Risk of corneal transplant rejection significantly reduced with Descemet's membrane endothelial keratoplasty. Ophthalmology 2012;119:536–540.

64 Dapena I, Ham L, Netuková M, et al: Incidence of early allograft rejection after Descemet membrane endothelial keratoplasty. Cornea 2011;30:1341–1345.

65 Steven P, Hos D, Heindl LM, et al: Immune reactions after DMEK, DSAEK and DALK. Klin Monbi Augenheilkd 2013;230:494–499.

66 Price FW Jr, Price MO: Descemet's stripping with endothelial keratoplasty in 200 eyes: early challenges and techniques to enhance donor adherence. J Cataract Refract Surg 2006;32:411–418.

67 Kruse FE, Schrehardt US, Tourtas T: Optimizing outcomes with Descemet's membrane endothelail keratoplasty. Curr Opin Ophthalmol 2014;25:325–334.

68 Studeny P, Farkas A, Vokrojova M, et al: Descemet membrane endothelial keratoplasty with a stromal rim (DMEK-S). Br J Ophthalmol 2010;94:909–914.

69 Pereira CDR, Guerra FP, Price FW Jr, et al: Descemet's membrane automated endothelial keratoplasty (DMAEK): visual outcomes and visual quality. Br J Ophthalmol 2011;95:951–954.

70 McCauley MB, Price FW Jr, Price MO: Descemet membrane automated endothelial keratoplasty: hybrid technique combining DSAEK stability with DMEK visual results. J Cataract Refract Surg 2009;35:1659–1664.

71 Busin M, Patel AK, Scorcia V, et al: Stromal support for Descemet's membrane endothelial keratoplasty. Ophthalmology 2010;117:2273–2277.

72 Yoeruek E, Bayyoud T, Hofmann J, et al: Comparison of pneumatic dissection and forceps dissection in Descemet membrane endothelial keratoplasty: histological and ultrastructural findings. Cornea 2012;31:920–925.

73 Venzano D, Pagani P, Randazzo N, et al: Descemet membrane air-bubbleseparation in donorcorneas. J Cataract Refract Surg 2010;36:2022–2027.

74 Kruse FE, Laaser K, Cursiefen C, et al: A stepwise approach to donor preparation and insertion increases safety and outcome of Descemet membrane endothelial keratoplasty. Cornea 2011;30:580–587.

75 Güell JL, Morral M, Gris O, et al: Bimanual technique for insertione graft in Descemet membrane endothelial keratoplasty. Cornea 2013;32:1521–1526.

76 McKee Y, Price MO, Gunderson L, et al: Rapid sequential endothelial keratoplasty with and without combined cataract extraction. J Cataract Refract Surg 2013;39:1372–1376.

77 Rock T, Bartz-Schmidt KU, Rock D, et al: [Refractive changes after Descemet membrane endothelial keratoplasty]. Ophthalmologe 2014;111:649–653.

78 Dapena I, Yeh RY, Baydoun L, et al: Potential causes of incomplete visual rehabilitation at 6 months postoperative after Descemet membrane endothelial keratoplasty. Am J Ophthalmol 2013;156:780–788.

79 van Dijk K, Parker J, Liarakis VS, et al: Incidence of irregular astigmatism eligible for contact lens fitting after Descemet membrane endothelial keratoplasty. J Cataract Refrac Surg 2013;39:1036–1046.

80 Liarakos VS, Dapena I, Ham L, et al: Intraocular graft unfolding techniques in Descemet membrane endothelial keratoplasty. JAMA Ophthalmol 2013;131:29–35.

81 Ham L, Dapena I, Moutsouris K, et al: Refractive change and stability after Descemet membrane endothelial keratoplasty. Effect of corneal dehydration-induced hyperopic shift on intraocular lens power calculation. J Cataract Refract Surg 2011;37:1455–1464.

82 Dapena I, Ham L, Droutsas K, et al: Learning curve in Descemet's membrane endothelial keratoplasty: first series of 135 consecutive cases. Ophthalmology 2011;118:2147–2154.

83 Heindl LM, Riss S, Laaser K, et al: Split cornea transplantation for 2 recipients – review of the first 100 consecutive patients. Am J Ophthalmol 2011;152:523–532.

84 Laaser K, Bachmann BO, Horn FK, et al: Descemet membrane endothelial keratoplasty combined with phacoemulsification and intraocular lens implantation: advanced triple procedure. Am J Ophthalmol 2012;154:47–55.

85 Tourtas T, Schlomberg J, Wessel JM, et al: Graft adhesion in Descemet membrane endothelial keratoplasty dependent on size of removal of host's Descemet membrane. JAMA Ophthalmol 2014;132:155–161.

86 Burkhart ZN, Feng MT, Price MO, et al: Handheld slit beam techniques to facilitate DMEK and DALK. Cornea 2013;32:722–724.

87 Dirisamer M, van Dijk K, Dapena I, et al: Prevention and management of graft detachment in descemet membrane endothelial keratoplasty. Arch Ophthalmol 2012;130:280–291.

88 Dapena I, Moutsouris K, Ham L, et al: Graft detachment rate. Ophthalmology 2010;117:847.

89 Laaser K, Bachmann BO, Horn FK, et al: Donor tissue culture conditions and outcome after Descemet membrane endothelial keratoplasty. Am J Ophthalmol 2011;151:1007–1018.

90 Gault JA, Raber IM: Repair of Descemet's membrane detachment with intracameral injection of 20% sulfur hexafluoride gas. Cornea 1996;15:483–489.

91 Mahmood MA, Teichmann KD, Tomey KF, et al: Detachment of Descemet's membrane. J Cataract Refract Surg 1998;24:827–833.

92 Thompson JT: Kinetics of intraocular gases. Disappearance of air, sulfur hexafluoride, and perfluoropropane after pars plana vitrectomy. Arch Ophthalmol 1989;107:687–691.

93 Lee DA, Wilson MR, Yoshizumi MO, et al: The ocular effects of gases when injected into the anterior chamber of rabbit eyes. Arch Ophthalmol 1991;109:571–575.

94 Mittra RA, Pollack JS, Dev S, et al: The use of topical aqueous suppressants in the prevention of postoperative intraocular pressure elevation after pars plana vitrectomy with long-acting gas tamponade. Ophthalmology 2000;107:588–592.

95 Chen PP, Thompson JT: Risk factors for elevated intraocular pressure after the use of intraocular gases in vitreoretinal surgery. Ophthalmic Surg Lasers 1997;28:37–42.

96 Liarakos VS, Ham L, Dapena I, et al: Endothelial keratoplasty for bullous keratopathy in eyes with an anterior chamber intraocular lens. J Cataract Refract Surg 2013;39:1835–1845.

97 Chaurasia S, Price FW Jr, Gunderson L, et al: Descemet's membrane endothelial keratopalsty: clinical results of single versus tripe procedures (combined with Cataract surgery). Ophthalmology 2014;121:454–458.

98 Musa FU, Cabrerizo J, Quilendrino R, et al: Outcomes of phacoemulsification after Descemet membrane endotelial keratoplasty. J Cataract Refract Surg 2013;39:836–840.

99 Yoeruek E, Bartz-Schmidt KU: Secondary Descemet membrane endothelial keratoplasty after failed primary Descemet membrane endothelial keratoplasty: clinical results. Cornea 2013;32:1414–1417.

José L. Güell
IMO. Instituto Microcirugia Ocular of Barcelona
Autonoma University of Barcelona
C/ Josep Mª Lladó, 3
ES-08035 Barcelona (Spain)
E-Mail guell@imo.es

Subject Index